THE COMMONWEALTH AND INTERNATIONAL LIBRARY
Joint Chairmen of the Honorary Editorial Advisory Board
SIR ROBERT ROBINSON, O.M., F.R.S., LONDON
DEAN ATHELSTAN SPILHAUS, MINNESOTA
Publisher: ROBERT MAXWELL, M.C., M.P.

A COURSE IN ORGANIC CHEMISTRY
General Editor: SIR ROBERT ROBINSON

Introduction to Steroid Chemistry

Introduction
to Steroid Chemistry

BY

J. R. HANSON, M.A., B.SC., PH.D., D.I.C., A.R.I.C.
Lecturer in Chemistry, University of Sussex

THE QUEEN'S AWARD
TO INDUSTRY 1966

PERGAMON PRESS
OXFORD · LONDON · EDINBURGH · NEW YORK
TORONTO · SYDNEY · PARIS · BRAUNSCHWEIG

Pergamon Press Ltd., Headington Hill Hall, Oxford
4 & 5 Fitzroy Square, London W.1
Pergamon Press (Scotland) Ltd., 2 & 3 Teviot Place, Edinburgh 1
Pergamon Press Inc., 44–01 21st Street, Long Island City, New York 11101
Pergamon of Canada Ltd., 207 Queen's Quay West, Toronto 1
Pergamon Press (Aust.) Pty. Ltd., 19A Boundary Street, Rushcutters Bay,
N.S.W. 2011
Pergamon Press S.A.R.L., 24 rue des Écoles, Paris 5e
Vieweg & Sohn GmbH, Burgplatz 1, Braunschweig

Filmset by The European Printing Corporation Limited, Dublin, Ireland
Printed in Great Britain by A. Wheaton & Co., Exeter

08 103759 7 (flexicover)
08 203759 0 (hard cover)

254927

Contents

v

Foreword

THE steroids form a group of compounds of immense biological importance. Consequently their chemistry has been the subject of intensive investigations with results whose ramifications have spread far beyond the bounds of steroid chemistry. It is fair to say that our knowledge of the conformational features of reactivity would be severely limited but for the investigation of the steroids. The same can be said of synthetic organic chemistry.

It is the aim of this short text to provide an introduction to the subject designed for the advanced undergraduate who is already familiar with general organic chemistry and the research worker who may be starting on a steroid problem. I hope it might also assist research workers in related subjects, particularly biochemistry, if they wished to obtain an introduction to present-day steroid chemistry.

There exist a number of specialist monographs in this field such as Fieser and Fieser's *Steroids,* Shoppee's *Chemistry of the Steroids* and Djerassi's *Steroid Reactions.* These serve as major works of reference and it is assumed that the reader will be able to turn to these authoritative texts for further reading. In addition, progress can be followed by consulting *The Chemical Society Annual Reports, Annual Reviews of Biochemistry,* and *Vitamins and Hormones.* At the end of each chapter a few review articles have been mentioned. These contain detailed information which expand particular points.

Finally my thanks are due to Miss Sue Wilson, who carefully typed the manuscript.

University of Sussex   J. R. H.
February 1967

CHAPTER 1

Introduction

THE steroids are a group of substances of both plant and animal origin possessing a characteristic tetracyclic backbone (1). They have been defined in a number of ways. Biogenetically they are a group of triterpenoid substances embodying six isopentenyl units. They may be distinguished from other – less important – groups of triterpene by the absence of three methyl groups. These features can be seen in a comparison of squalene (2), lanosterol (3) and the best known of the steroids, cholesterol (4). Closer inspection of the formulae of the tetracyclic triterpene, lanosterol and the

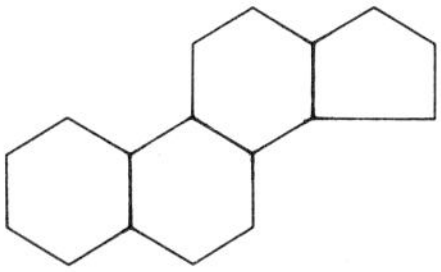

1

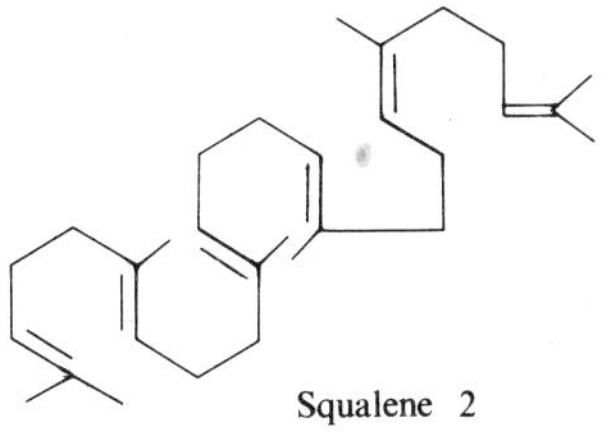

Squalene 2

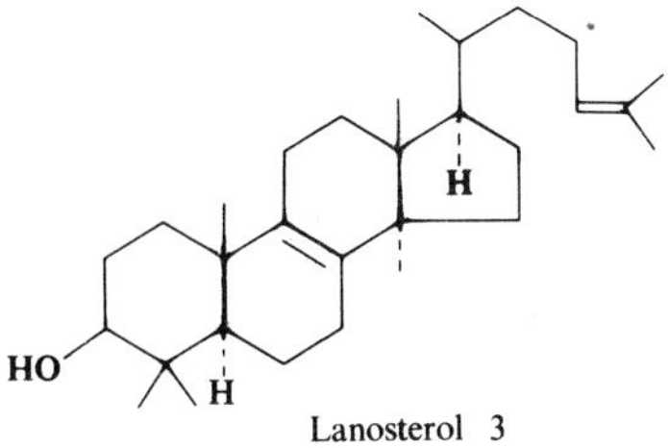

Lanosterol 3

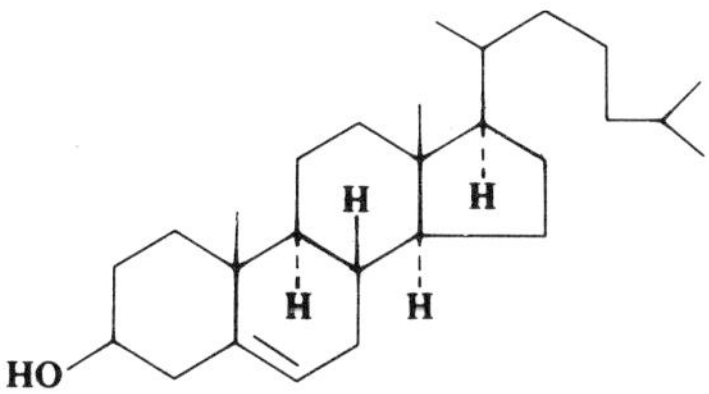

Cholesterol 4

steroid, cholesterol shows that the characteristic methylation pattern involves a rearrangement of the pattern in squalene.

Amongst the steroids are substances of very considerable medicinal importance. These include the sex hormones such as oestrone (5), androsterone (6) and progesterone (7), the adrenocortical hormones such as cortisone (8), the antirachitic vitamin — vitamin D_2 (9) — and the cardiac glycosides which are sugar derivatives of steroids such as digitoxigenin (10). Recently a steroidal antibiotic, fusidic acid (11), has been marketed. Related to these compounds are a wide variety of analogues that have been introduced into therapy to correct hormone deficiencies, as anabolic agents, to alleviate rheumatoid arthritis, various skin conditions, and more recently as oral contraceptives. The bile-acids occur as conjugates with amino-acids. Thus glycocholic acid, $RCONH \cdot CH_2 \cdot CO_2H$, contains a steroid fragment, cholic acid (12) linked as an amide to glycine. The sodium salts of these conjugates facilitate the absorption of fat from the intestine.

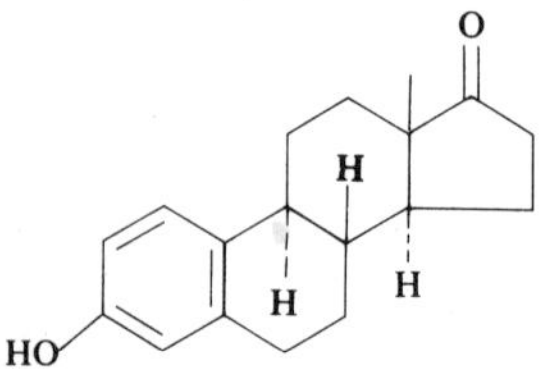

Oestrone   5

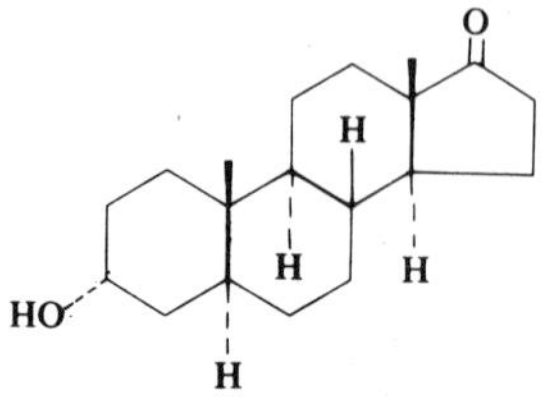

Androsterone   6

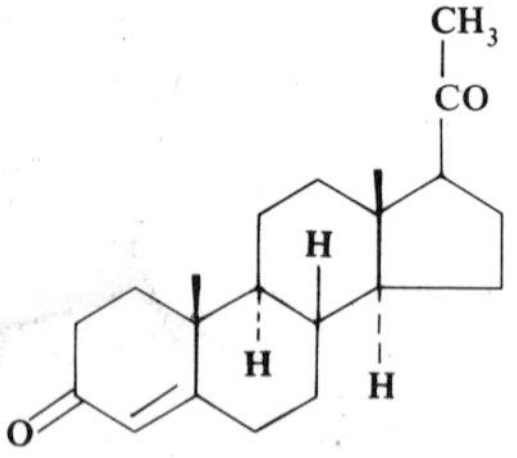

Progesterone   7

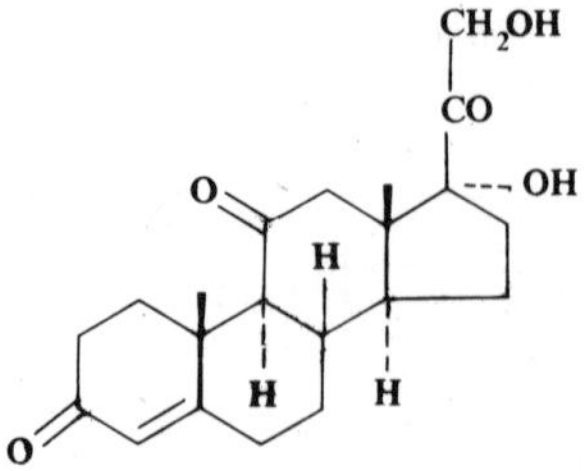

Cortisone   8

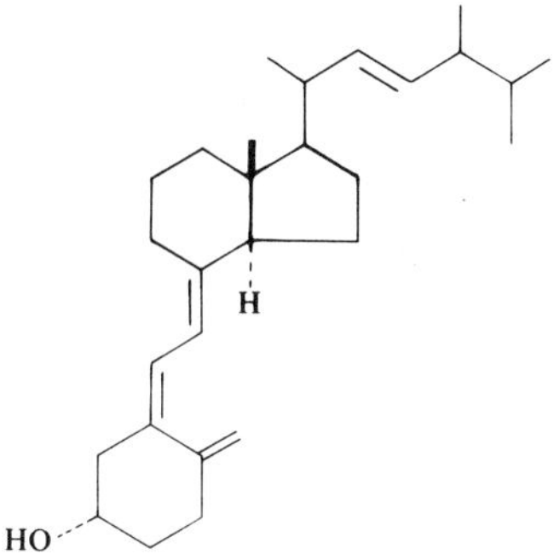

Vitamin D$_2$ 9

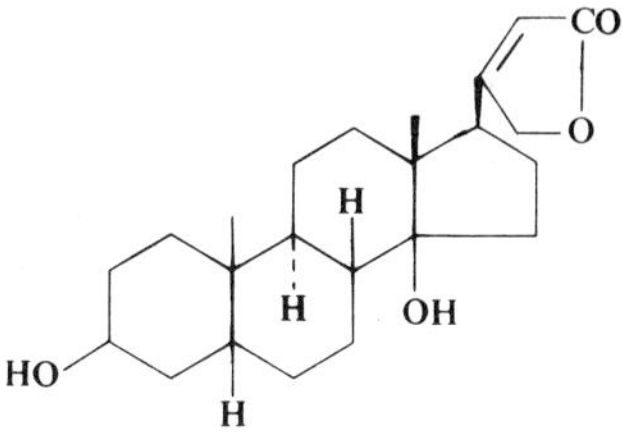

Digitoxigenin   10

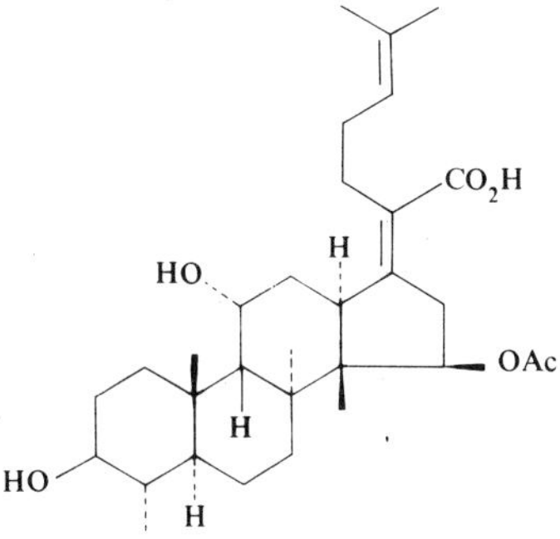

Fusidic Acid   11

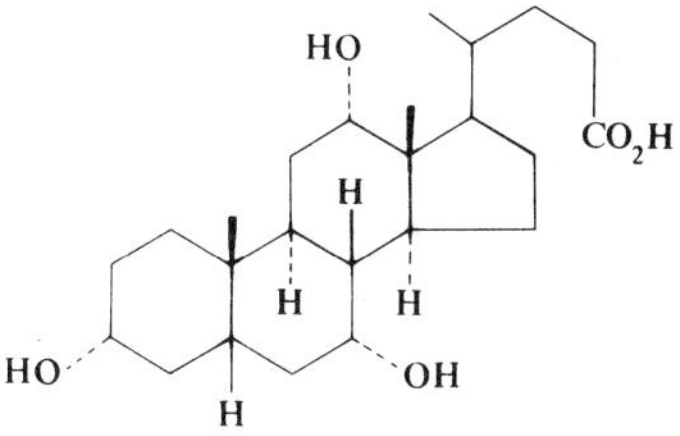

Cholic Acid   12

A number of alkaloids such as solanidine (13) whose glycoside solanine occurs in potato sprouts, possess a steroidal structure, whilst insect hormones such as ecdysone (14) also belong to this class. These examples serve to illustrate the variety of steroid structures. However, throughout, the common backbone is clear.

The steroids are numbered as in (15). In drawing formulae the convention is used in which a dotted or broken line represents the α-configuration for a substituent (i.e. it lies below the general plane of the ring) whilst a solid or thickened line denotes the β-configuration (i.e. the substituent lies above

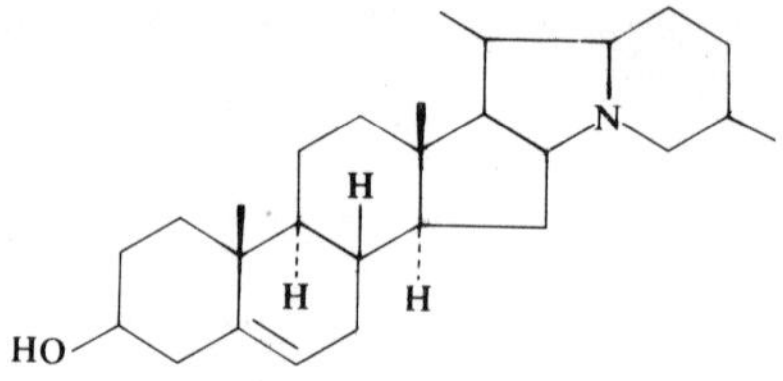

Solanidine 13

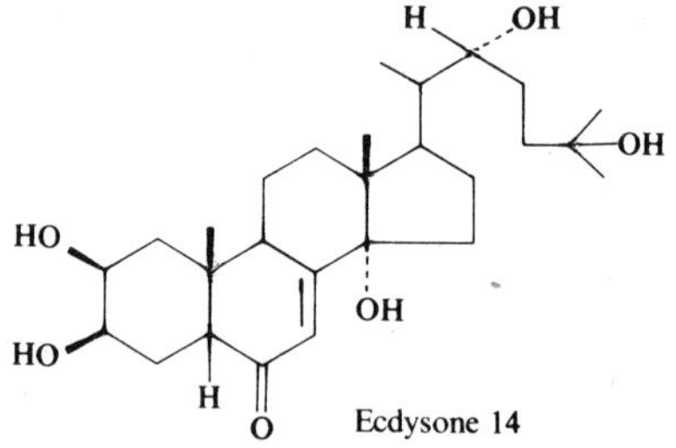

Ecdysone 14

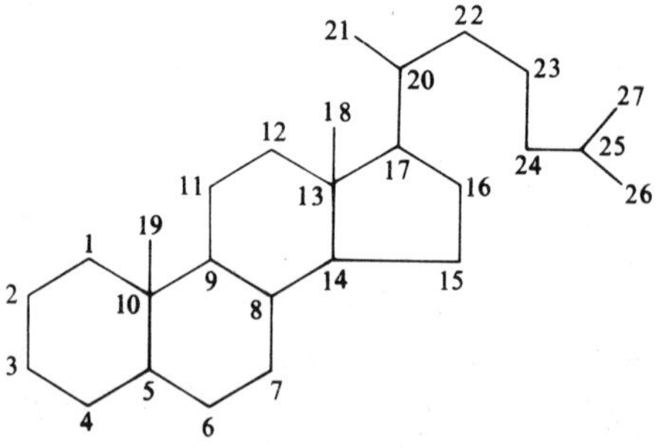

15

the general plane of the ring). Fortunately this convention represents the absolute configuration. Where the configuration is unknown this is indicated by the Greek letter ξ (xi) and in the formula by a wavy line.

The common parent hydrocarbons are described as follows:

	5α − series	5β − series
R = H	5α − Androstane	5β − Androstane
R = C₂H₅	5α − Pregnane	5β − Pregnane
R =	5α − Cholane	5β − Cholane
R =	5α − Cholestane	5β − Cholestane

The name "gonane" is used for the hydrocarbon lacking both methyl groups and a side chain whilst the name oestrane applies to the saturated hydrocarbon lacking the methyl group at C-10 and the side chain at C-17.

There are two A/B ring fusions which occur naturally. These are the "*cis*" fusion of the bile-acids and the "*trans*" fusion of, for example, androsterone. In the older literature the *cis* fusion of 5β-cholestane is often described as the "coprostane" system and the name "cholestane" retained for the *trans* fusion. Definitive rules such as the I.U.P.A.C. 1957 Rules for the Nomenclature of Steroids have been produced for the systematic description of steroids.† These rules are followed by the major publications. However, for convenience, structural formulae are very widely used.

The steroids have been known for over 150 years. Although cholesterol was described as early as 1812 and the bile-acid, cholic acid in 1828, the correct structure of cholesterol (4) was

† See *Handbook for Chemical Society Authors*, The Chemical Society, London, 1960.

not proposed until 1932. The investigation of the steroids falls historically into a number of phases. Prior to the work of Windaus and Diels which began in 1903, the study of cholesterol, and the bile-acids, was concerned with their analysis and characterization. Thus cholesterol, which was isolated from gall stones, was shown to be a secondary alcohol and as it formed a dibromide, to contain one double bond. Analyses eventually led to the $C_{27}H_{40}O$ formulation for cholesterol.

The relationship of the double bond and hydroxyl group became apparent from a number of degradations. Thus oxidative cleavage of ring A with sodium hypobromite gave a dicarboxylic acid (16) known as the Diels' acid. This acid retained the double bond of cholesterol although in a modified chemical environment. On the other hand nitration of the double bond of cholesterol and reduction of the nitro compound led to a 6-ketone. This then permitted the oxidative cleavage of the ring containing the double bond to form a dicarboxylic acid (17). One of these carboxyls lactonized onto the ring A hydroxyl indicating that these functions lay in adjacent rings.

Diels' Acid   16

17

The proximity of the hydroxyl group and double bond was also indicated by the formation of cholest-4-en-3-one on oxidation of cholesterol. However, conclusive evidence for double-bond migration during this oxidation involved the isolation of the intermediate cholest-5-en-3-one. This was not achieved until after the structure of cholesterol was proven. The method used involved protection of the double bond as its dibromide, controlled oxidation with sodium dichromate and followed by debromination with zinc dust.

Reduction of the double bond by bacterial means gave the *cis* fused isomer, coprostanol, whilst chemical reduction gave the *trans* fused cholestanol. The relationship between the two

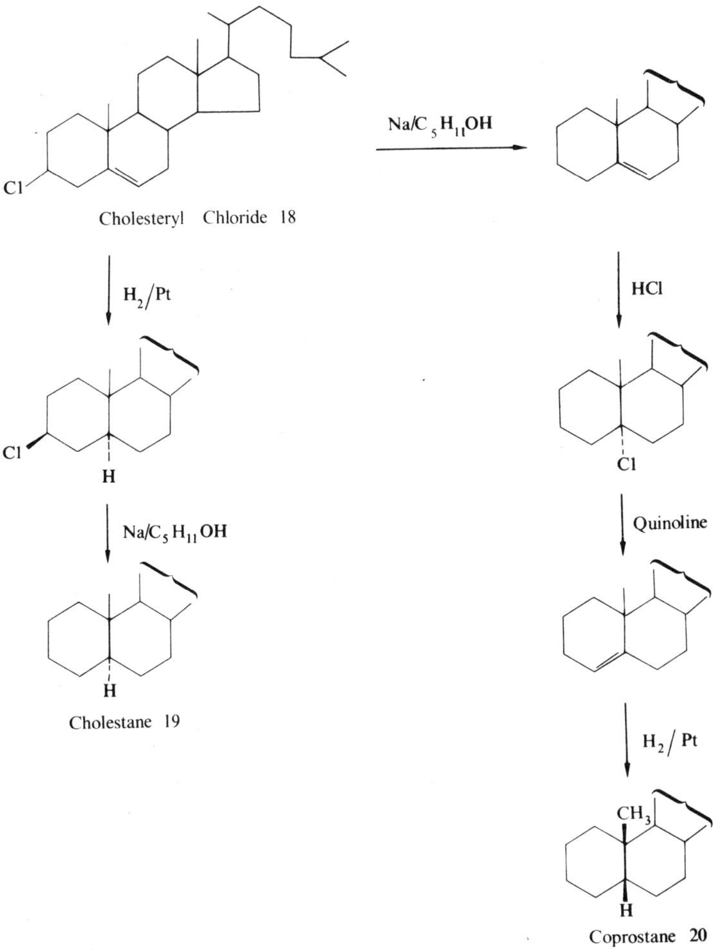

Cholesteryl Chloride 18

Na/C$_5$H$_{11}$OH

H$_2$/Pt

Cl
H

Na/C$_5$H$_{11}$OH

Cholestane 19

HCl

Cl

Quinoline

H$_2$/Pt

CH$_3$
H

Coprostane 20

was established by the degradation of cholesteryl chloride (18) to the parent hydrocarbons, cholestane (19) and coprostane (20). This degradation shows a number of features. These are: firstly, the 5α-diaxial addition of hydrogen chloride; secondly, the formation of the Δ^4-double bond by attack of the slightly less-hindered 4β-proton and thirdly the difference between catalytic hydrogenation of a Δ^4- and Δ^5-double bond.

Cleavage of the side-chain of cholesterol gave methyl iso-hexyl ketone by attack at a tertiary centre. Oxidation of coprostane (5β-cholstane) led to an alternative mode of cleavage and the formation of cholanic acid (21) — a degradation product of the bile acids. Hence structural evidence obtained from the study of the bile acids by Windaus and Wieland was applied to the structure of cholesterol. The study of the bile acids was facilitated by the fact that they contain oxygen functions in three of the four rings.

Cholanic Acid

21

The determination of the size of these rings during the 1920's involved the application of Blanc's rule. This rule states that pyrolysis of $1:5$-dicarboxylic acids leads to the formation of anhydrides whilst $1:6$-dicarboxylic acids form ketones (cyclo-pentanones). For example oxidation of cholestanol gave the $2:3$-dicarboxylic acid. Pyrolysis of this gave a cyclopentanone — A-norcholestanone (22) and thus ring A was six-membered. This degradation was extended to desoxycholic acid (26) and resulted in the stepwise cleavage of each ring. Ring B was thus

22

shown to be six-membered. In this degradation the heavily substituted ring C unfortunately was not converted to a cyclopentanone but formed an anhydride. Hence it was originally thought to be five-membered. This limitation of Blanc's rule became apparent in 1932 when a 6:7-dicarboxylic acid retaining both rings A and C gave an anhydride and hence also failed to conform to the rule.

Access to ring D was obtained by degradation of the side-chain. This procedure (23) due to Barbier and Wieland, involves the Grignard reaction of phenyl magnesium bromide with an ester of, for example, cholanic acid. Oxidation of the resultant tertiary alcohol led to the nor-carboxylic acid. Eventual cleavage of ring D showed it to be five-membered.

Barbier — Wieland Degradation 23

In 1927 and 1928 the Nobel prize was awarded to Wieland and Windaus. Wieland, in summarizing the work up to that time, proposed a tentative formula (24) for desoxycholic acid. This contained a five-membered ring C and a carbon atom which was common to three rings. However, in 1932 X-ray measurements made by Bernal on ergosterol indicated that the steroid molecule was long and flat as opposed to the thick structure implicit in (24). The significance of an earlier observation made in 1927 by Diels then became apparent. Dehydrogenation of cholesterol gave chrysene and a hydro-carbon which was subsequently shown to be (25). Consequently a perhydrochrysene formula for desoxycholic acid was pro-posed by Rosenheim and King. This was modified to the accepted structure for desoxycholic acid (26) by Rosenheim and King and by Wieland and Dane in papers which appeared within a few weeks of each other in the autumn of 1932.

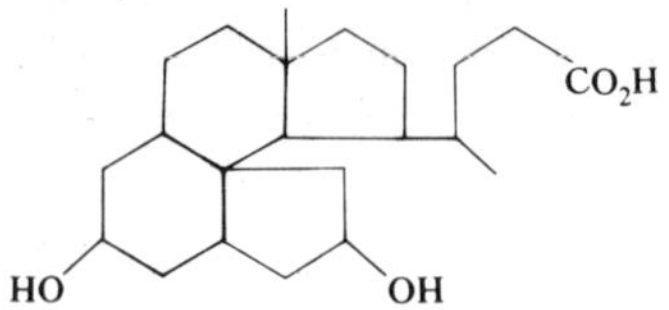

CO_2H

HO   OH

+ C_2H_4

24

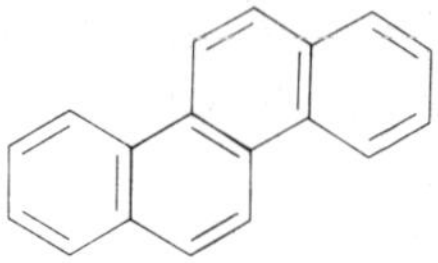

Chrysene

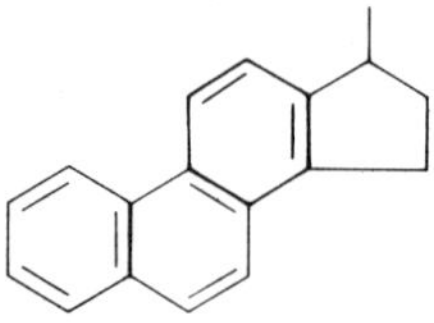

Diels' Hydrocarbon

25

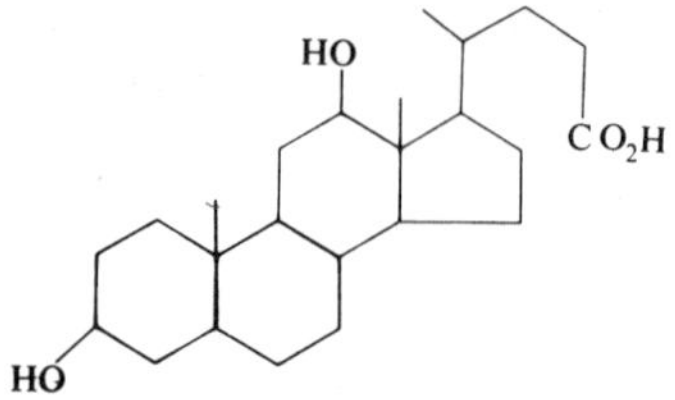

HO

CO_2H

HO

Desoxycholic Acid

26

The location of the methyl groups on the perhydrophenan-threne backbone was established by stepwise degradation of ring A and of ring C to the appropriate tertiary acids. The position of the side-chain evident from the Barbier–Wieland degradation, was also revealed by dehydrogenation of desoxy-cholic acid to give methyl cholanthrene which was synthesized.

The stereochemistry of the various ring fusions was assigned on the basis of stability relationships. Thus one of the bile acids, hyodesoxycholic acid (27), was oxidized to a diketone.

This behaved as a *cis* decalone and was isomerized to a *trans* fused system and hence the coprostane (5β-cholestane) series was *cis* fused. Further evidence in support of this came later from the formation of 3:9-oxides. Displacement of the allylic chloride (28) gave a 3:9-oxide (29) the formation of which requires not only a 3α-hydroxyl group but also a *cis* A/B fusion. On the other hand the stability to base of the 7-ketones indicated a *trans* B/C fusion. The *trans* stereochemistry of the C/D fusion was apparent from the cleavage of ring C to form the tricarboxylic acid (30). This underwent isomerization to a *cis* acid prior to the formation of an anhydride. This chemical evidence received support from X-ray measurements.

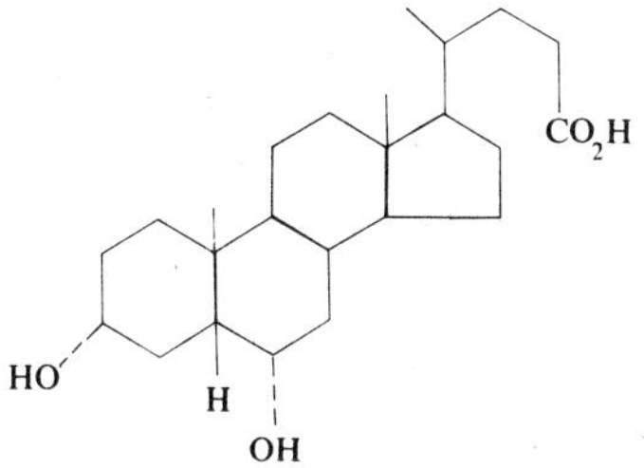

Hyodesoxycholic Acid 27

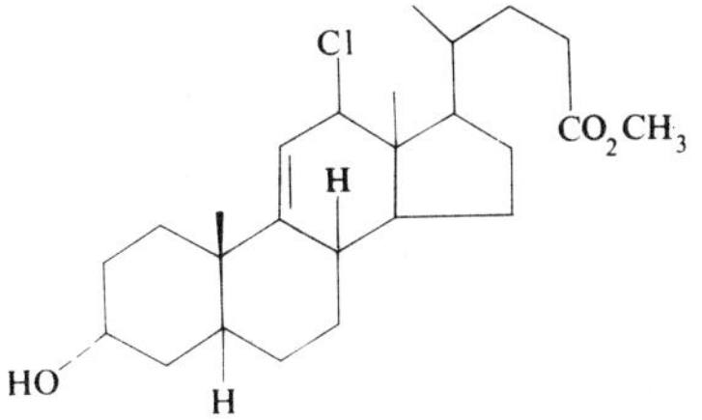

28

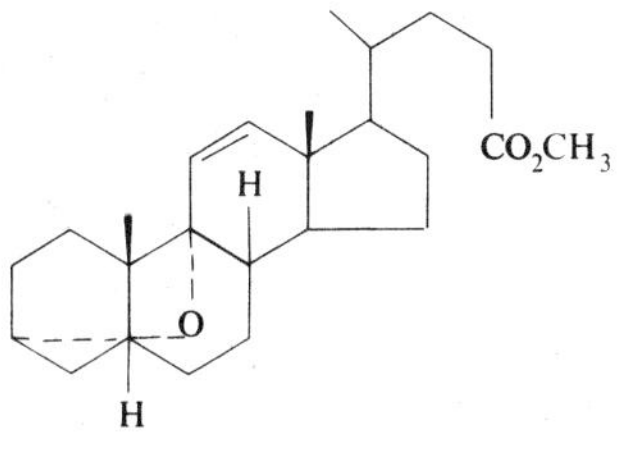

29

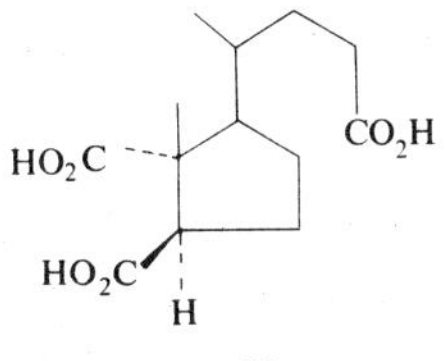

30

The late 1920's and 1930's saw the establishment of a number of bioassay techniques which led to the isolation of biologically active steroids. One of the most important of these was the antirachitic vitamin D. Studies on rickets induced in rats indicated that irradiation of the phytosterol component of food produced an antirachitic principle. The component which on irradiation formed vitamin D_2 was eventually isolated and shown to be ergosterol (31). The structure of vitamin D_2 (32) was finally established in 1936. X-ray analysis of the 4-iodo-5-nitrobenzoate showed that it possessed the transoid stereochemistry of the diene. The photochemical and thermal relationship of vitamin D_2 (calciferol) to ergosterol, lumisterol, precalciferol and tachysterol is discussed on p. 74.

Ergosterol 31   Vitamin D$_2$ 32

This period also saw the important discovery of the sex hormones each isolation following fairly rapidly from the development of convenient methods of bioassay. Three groups of steroidal sex hormone are now recognized. They are the oestrogens, the progestogens and the androgens. Oestrone (33) the best known of the oestrogenic ovarian hormones, was isolated in 1929 from pregnancy urine. Its structure and that of the related oestriol (34) were proposed in 1932. These hormones are characterized by an aromatic ring A with a phenolic hydroxyl group. It is this feature which distinguishes their chemistry and permits them to be separated from other urinary steroids. Whereas the oestrogens are associated with the onset of oestrus and the changes in the cell structure of the vaginal epithelium, the progestogens are associated with the formation of the corpus lutea and the maintenance of pregnancy. Progesterone (35) was isolated in 1934 in small amount (20 mg) from 625-kg sow ovaries representing 50,000 animals. The presence of an $\alpha\beta$-unsaturated ketone was demonstrated by its ultraviolet spectrum in one of the early applications of physical methods to natural product problems. Its structure was proven by partial synthesis from pregnane diol (3β-pregnane-3α, 20α-diol).

The androgens are compounds which are associated with the development of the male sex organs and secondary

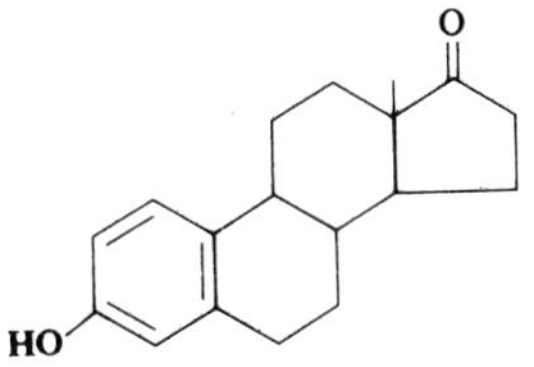

Oestrone   33

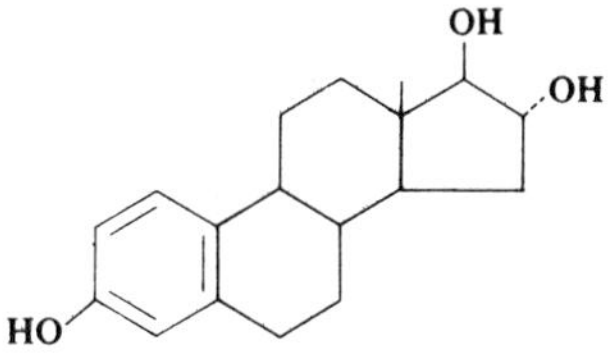

Oestriol   34

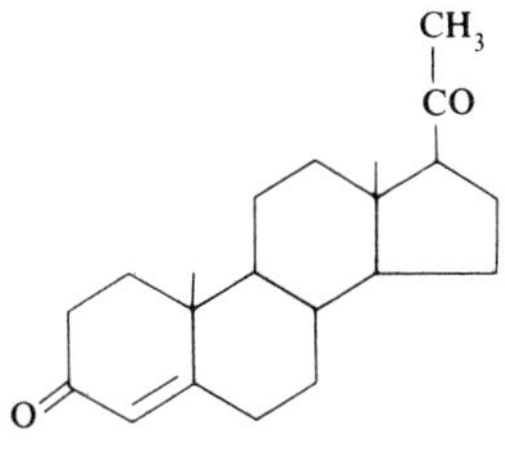

Progesterone   35

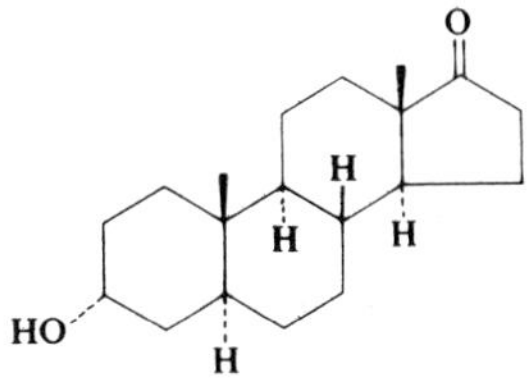

Androsterone   36

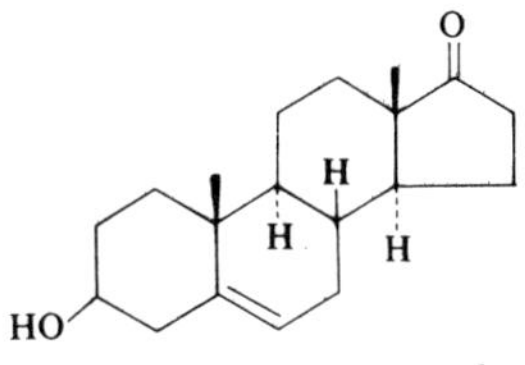

Dehydroepiandrosterone   37

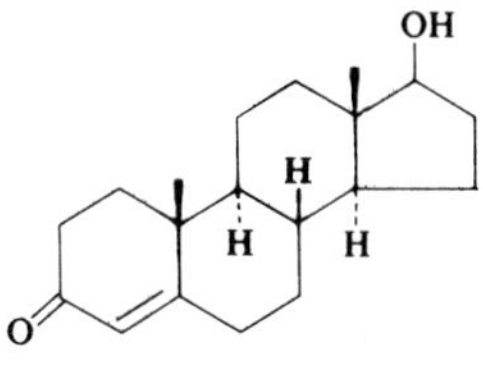

Testosterone   38

sexual characteristics. Androsterone (36) isolated in 1931, dehydroepiandrosterone (37) and testosterone (38) are the best known members of this group. The development of the Girard reagents facilitated the separation of ketonic components from extracts in this work. Girard's reagent, $[(CH_3)_3N \cdot CH_2 \cdot CO \cdot NH \cdot NH_2]Cl^-$, functions by forming a water-soluble hydrazone which may be separated from the non-ketonic material. Acid hydrolysis of the hydrazone then regenerates the ketone.

The adrenocortical hormones represent another series of steroidal hormones isolated from 1936 onwards. These hormones excreted by the adrenal glands, control the electrolyte balance in the body (mineralocorticoid activity) and promote carbohydrate synthesis and the deposit of glycogen in the liver (glucocorticoid acitivity). The structure of cortisone (39) was proposed in 1938. During the later war years because of its scarcity from natural sources (75 mg cortisone was isolated from the adrenal glands of 20,000 cattle), considerable effort was directed at the partial synthesis of cortisone from more readily available steroids such as desoxycholic acid. The discovery of the action of cortisone in the treatment of rheumatoid arthritis in 1949 stimulated a great deal of research to find workable routes to the cortical hormones. These led not only to the partial synthesis of cortisone but also the synthesis of a number of analogues. The starting materials for these syntheses involve either the bile acids or plant steroids such as stigmasterol (40) or the sapogenin, diosgenin (41). In the case of diosgenin the spiroketal side-chain is degraded first to 16-dehydropregnenolone acetate which can then be converted through Beckmann rearrangement of the oxime to the androstane series. Alternatively the cortical hormones were produced by modification of the side-chain, introduction of oxygen at C-11 and formation of an $\alpha\beta$-unsaturated ketone on ring A. Some of these steps are outlined in Chapter 5. In 1954 a hormone aldosterone with very high mineral corticoid activity was isolated from adrenal glands.

Although very little material was available the structure (42) which has subsequently been confirmed by synthesis, was assigned to aldosterone. The pre-war period also saw the investigation of a number of other naturally occurring steroids. The cardenolides form an important group of steroidal glycosides capable in very small amounts, of stimulating the heart muscles. A well-known source is the foxglove *Digitalis*

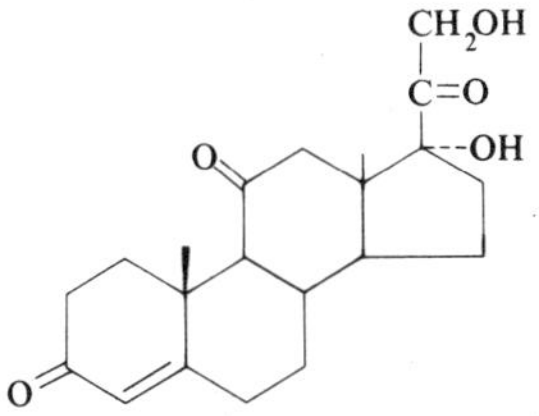

Cortisone 39

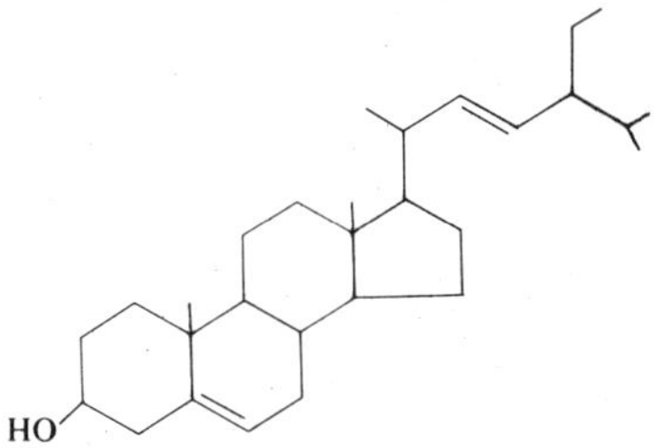

Stigmasterol 40

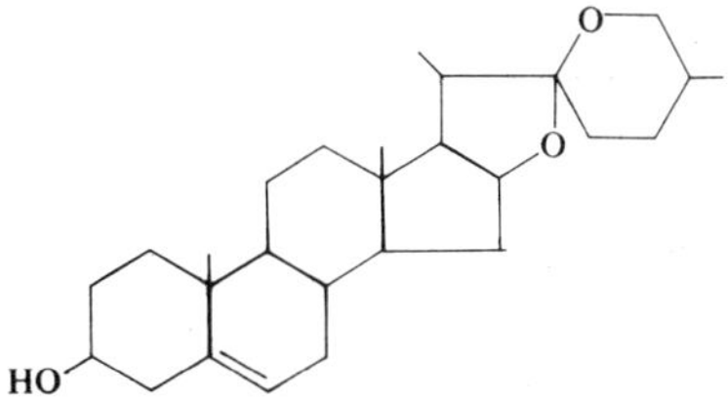

Diosgenin 41

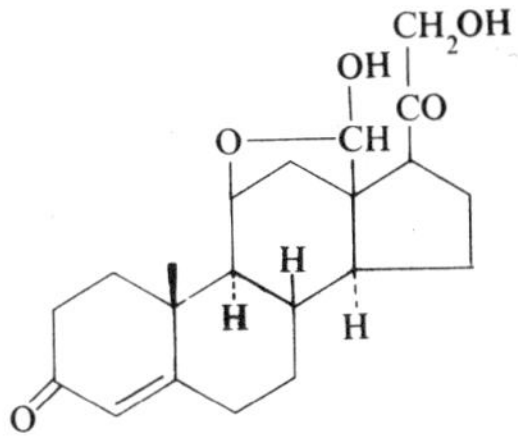

Aldosterone 42

purpurea in which one of the aglycones is digitoxigenin (43). The sugar residues are attached to position 3. Much of the early structural work from 1923 onwards was carried out with strophanthidin (44). In the event this proved an unfortunate choice since strophanthidin, as a consequence of its tertiary hydroxyl at C-5 and angular aldehyde group, undergoes a number of dehydration, rearrangement and lactone formation reactions which are not shown by digitoxigenin.

The characteristic feature of the aglycones is the butenolide ($\alpha\beta$-unsaturated lactone) grouping and the *cis* C/D ring junction with a 14β-hydroxyl group. The side-chain distinguishes them from the bufadienolides such as scillaren A which possess an α-pyrone in place of the butenolide ring. The toad venoms also belong to this group of steroids.

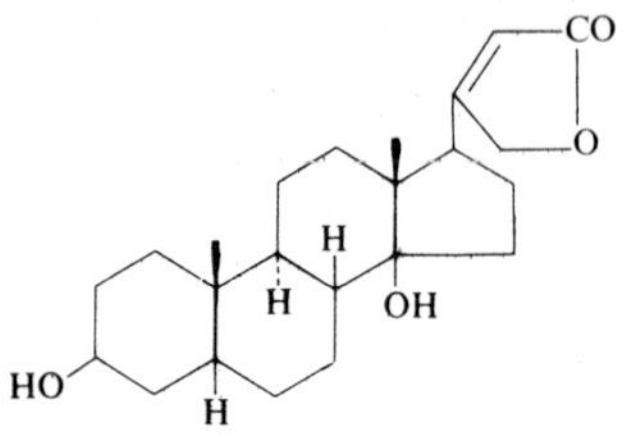

Digitoxigenin 43

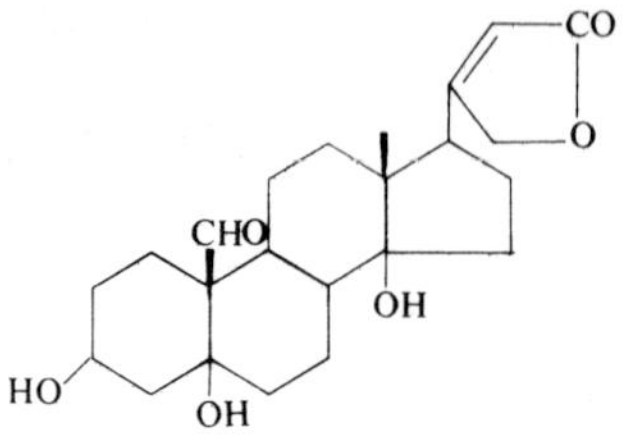

Strophanthidin   44

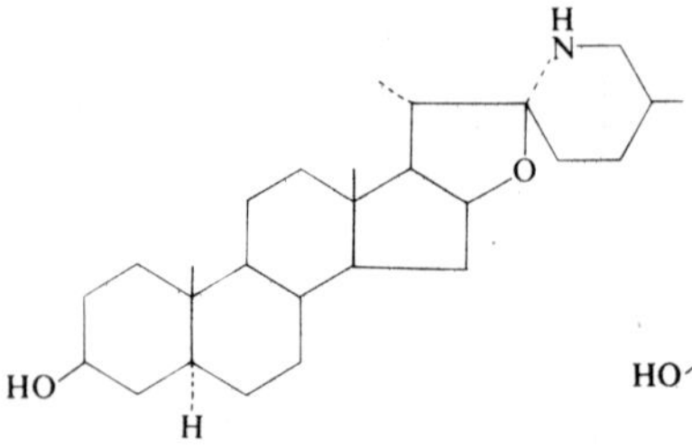

Tomatidine 45

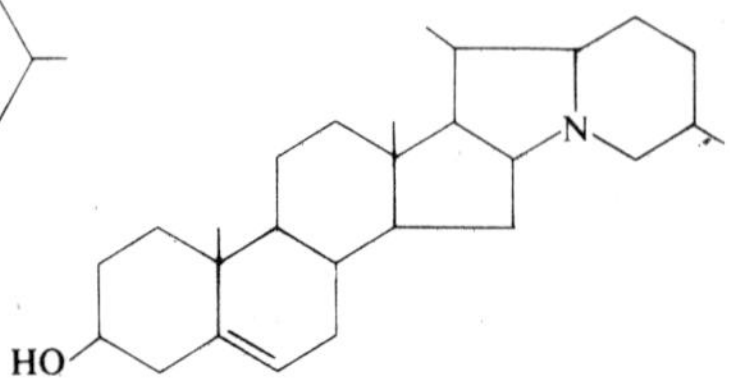

Solanidine 46

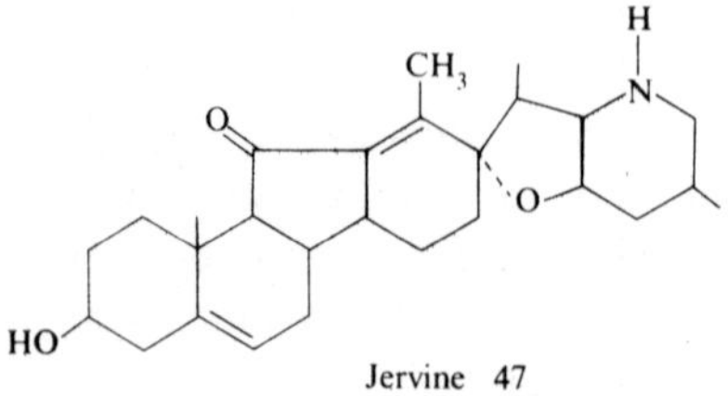

Jervine 47

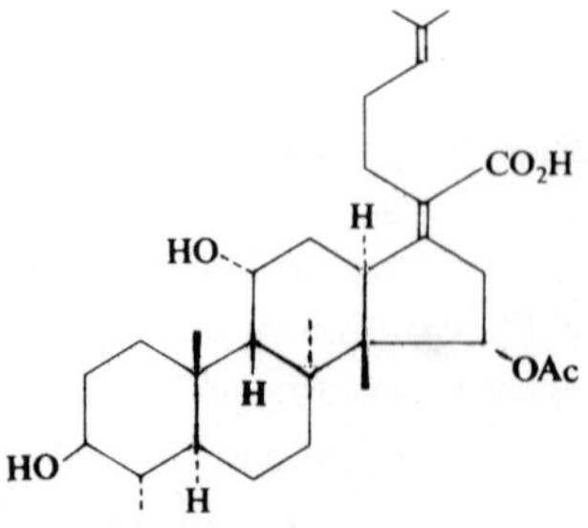

Fusidic Acid 48

Another large group of plant glycosides have a marked surface active action and are known as the saponins (aglycones = sapogenins). The characteristic structural feature of this group of steroids exemplified by diosgenin (41) is the spiroketal side-chain. Although digitogenin (from Digitalis) had been the subject of a number of earlier investigations the main stimulus for research in this field was to find suitable compounds for transformation into the steroidal hormones. A similar system involving, however, a nitrogen atom is found in the steroidal alkaloids such as tomatidine (45) and solanidine (46) isolated from *Solanum* species. Modification of rings C and D is found in the hypotensive *Veratrum* alkaloids such as jervine (47).

A number of compounds related to the steroids have been isolated from fungal sources. Although the majority such as the polyporenic acids are strictly tetracyclic triterpenes there are a few steroidal antibiotics. Fusidic acid (48) is one of these that has become commercially available.

The total synthesis of the steroids was begun during the later 1930's. The synthesis of equilenin (49) which contains only two centres of asymmetry was completed in 1939 whilst

Equilenin 49

a synthesis of oestrone was reported in 1947. The first total syntheses of non-aromatic steroids completed in Oxford and Harvard were reported almost simultaneously in 1951. The increasing control over the stereochemical consequences of chemical reactions which has been developed in the last 15 years has permitted many different approaches to the total synthesis of the steroids. Improvements in the synthesis of the oestrogenic hormones has enabled some methods to be worked economically on an industrial scale. These topics are discussed in more detail in Chapter 5.

Complementing the chemical work of structural determination and synthesis, the biochemistry of the steroids has been the subject of many investigations. Much of the pathway in the biosynthesis and subsequent metabolism of cholesterol is known. The advent of tracer techniques have enabled many of the steps to be clarified both in the synthetic sequence and in transformation of the steroids to the bile acids and various hormones. The biosynthesis of the steroids is discussed in Chapter 6.

5α - cholestane Trans fused A/B 50

5β-cholestane Cis fused   A/B 51

The study of the chemistry of the steroids was facilitated by three important developments in general chemistry. The first was the application of chromatographic techniques, the second the development of spectroscopic techniques and the third the understanding of the stereochemical consequences of reactions.

The steroid framework provides a relatively rigid ring system in which the axial and equatorial bonds can be clearly distinguished (50) and (51). Furthermore, axial and equatorial epimers are usually separable and differ in their rotation, infrared and n.m.r. spectra. Hence the relative proportion and rate of formation of isomers generated in an experiment may be determined. The conformational analysis of elimination and substitution reactions at various centres on rings A and B, the bromination of ketones, the oxidation of alcohols and the addition reactions of olefins has been studied in detail. The generalizations proposed by Barton, and many other workers since 1950, based on work in the steroid series have been extended to many other fields of organic chemistry. The conformational analysis of steroid reactions forms the subject of Chapter 3.

CHAPTER 2

Application of
Physical Methods to Steroid Chemistry

THE relative conformational rigidity and variety of known compounds have made the steroids a valuable subject for study by physical methods. The detailed application of spectroscopy to this series has led to structural and stereochemical correlations which in turn have proved their value in the elucidation of other problems. It is out of place to describe either the theoretical development of these methods or general instrumental techniques. Indeed we assume the reader has some knowledge of these. Admirable descriptions are available in general and specialized textbooks which are listed, together with some review articles, at the end of the chapter.

2.1. APPLICATIONS OF ULTRAVIOLET
SPECTROSCOPY

The application of ultraviolet spectroscopy to steroidal problems has a long history. There are two main types of aliphatic conjugated chromophore with which we are concerned—namely dienes and $\alpha\beta$-unsaturated ketones. The first of these involves the electronic transition of a bonding π-electron to an antibonding π-orbital of the diene system ($\pi-\pi^*$ transitions), whilst the second involves the transfer of an electron from the π-orbital of an olefin to the π-system of the ketone with which it is conjugated—an electron transfer (E.T.) band. The extensive number of minor variations on the parent chromophore that are possible within the steroidal framework led to a series of empirical correlations which are summarized by the Woodward–Fieser rules. These rules in turn have received application far beyond the bounds of steroid chemistry.

In essence the Woodward–Fieser rules state that the position of the main absorption band [λ_{max}] is made up of two components. The first is due to the parent chromophore whilst the second takes account of auxochromes such as alkyl substituents, ring systems and solvent interactions. The sum of these leads to a calculated value of λ_{max} which should correspond to within a few mμ to that observed.

Dienes

There are two major types of diene chromophore. The first of these possesses a transoid and the second a cisoid conformation. Cyclic systems then fall into the two categories of heteroannular dienes analogous to the transoid series and homoannular dienes analogous to the cisoid series. The Woodward rules may then be summarized as follows:

(i) each alkyl substituent attached to the diene chromophore produces an increment of 5 mμ towards longer wavelength,

(ii) each exocyclic double bond produces a further increment of 5 mμ.

Thus the predicted diene absorption maximum can be arrived at.

TABLE 1. DIENE ABSORPTION

Parent:	Heteroannular dienes 214	Homoannular dienes 253
Increments:	Further double bond	30
	Alkyl substituent	5
	Exocyclic component	5
	Total	mμ

These calculations may be exemplified by cholesta-4,6-diene (1) and ergosterol (2).

Cholesta-4,6-diene (1)

Heteroannular parent	214
Alkyl substituents 3×5	15
Exocyclic component	5
λ_{max}(calc)	234 mμ
λ_{max}(obs)	234 mμ

Ergosterol (2)

Homoannular parent	253
Alkyl substituents 4×5	20
Exocyclic component 2×5	10
λ_{max}(calc)	283 mμ
λ_{max}(obs)	282 mμ

Although these rules predict with fair accuracy the position of the main absorption, certain cyclic systems give rise to a group of subsidiary bands which are valuable for diagnostic purposes. Thus a number of steroidal homoannular-5,7-dienes show two additional peaks appearing *ca.* 10 mμ on either side

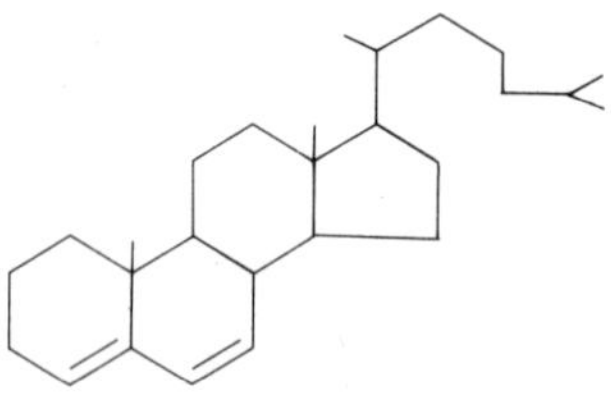

1

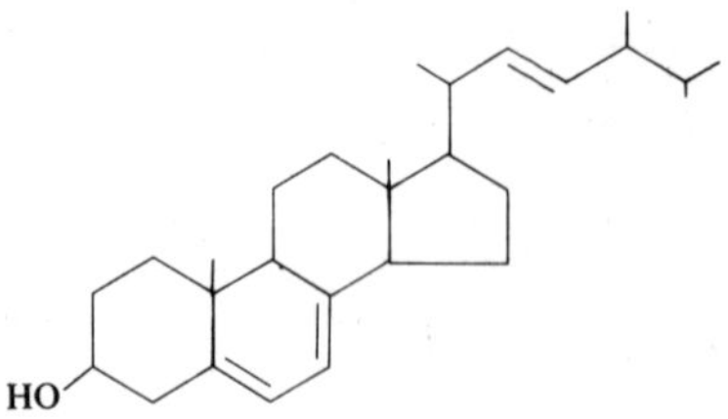

2

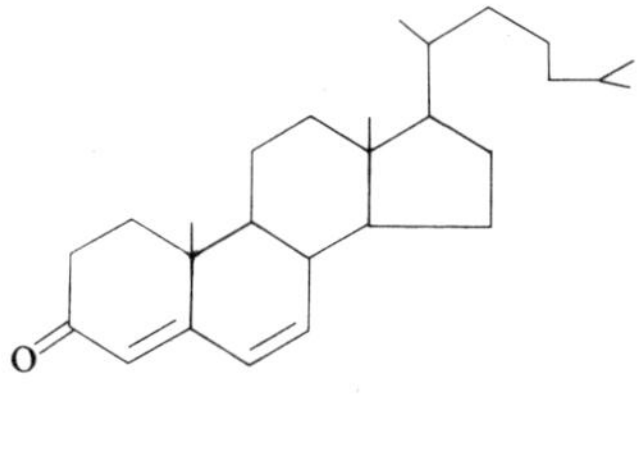

3

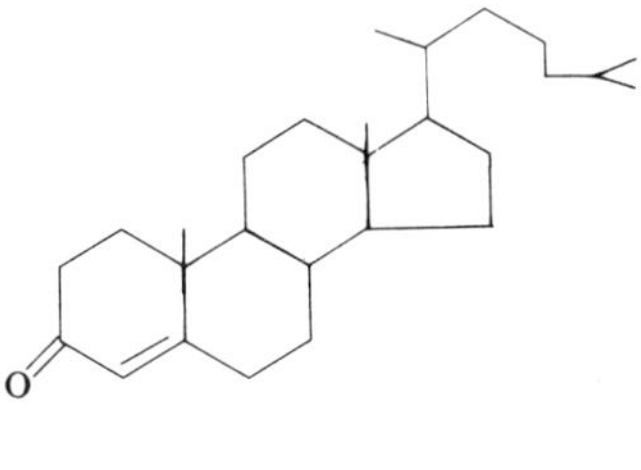

4

of the principle peak. In the case of heteroannular 7:9 (11)-dienes a similar fine structure can be used to distinguish between two possible naturally occurring *trans* C/D fusions of the lanostane and euphane series.

$\alpha\beta$-Unsaturated ketones

The predicted position of the absorption maxima for the electron transfer bands of $\alpha\beta$-unsaturated ketones can again be reliably calculated using Woodward rules.

TABLE 2. UNSATURATED KETONE ABSORPTION

Parent:	$\alpha\beta$-unsaturated ketone	215 mμ
Increments:	Further double bond	30
	Alkyl substituents α	10
	β	12
	γ, δ, etc.	18
	Hydroxyl substituents α	35
	β	30
	Exocyclic component	5
	Total	mμ

The calculations may be exemplified as follows:

Cholesta-4,6-diene-3-one (3)

λ_{max} Parent	215
Extending double bond	30
β substituent	12
δ substituent	18
Exocyclic component	5
λ_{max} (calc)	280
λ_{max} (obs)	284 mμ

Cholest-4-en-3-one (4)

λ_{max} Parent	215
β-substituents	24
Exocyclic component	5
λ_{max} (calc)	244 mμ
λ_{max} (obs)	241 mμ

The position of the parent chromophore reflects the ring size (five-membered-enone parent is at 205 mμ). Not unexpectedly as this transition involves the carbonyl oxygen which can form a site of solvation in the molecule, the final position of the λ_{max} is solvent dependent. By definition the calculated values are given in ethanol and a correction ranging from −8 mμ (water) to +11 mμ (cyclohexane) applied for the different solvents. If the olefinic component of a dienone belongs to a homoannular diene rather than a heteroannular diene (a $\Delta^{8(9),11}$-7-one rather than a $\Delta^{3,5}$-7-one) then a further 39 mμ homodiene increment is also added. The predicted values for cross-conjugated systems, present in enediones and other more complicated chromophores, show a much poorer degree of agreement and are less-useful correlations. However, such systems often show a characteristic multiple absorption and if the appropriate model system is available then a structural comparison can be made. A further feature which may modify the position of the major E.T. band (and also the weak n–π^* transition) is the interaction of the p-electrons of a γ-substituent. These effects which are found with halogen and oxygen substituents, are obviously dependent upon conformation.

Other absorptions

The clinical importance of many steroids has led to a considerable effort to determine the presence of minute amounts in urine and blood samples. Methods usually involve extraction and some partial purification followed by the application of a colour reaction under defined conditions which permit quantitative spectroscopy. For example, the Liebermann–Burchard colour reaction with chloroform, acetic anhydride and sulphuric acid has been used to estimate "blood" cholesterol, whilst other methods such as the Zimmerman reaction with *m*-dinitrobenzene have been used to estimate 17-keto steroids. These methods may define the presence of a particular chromophore but only rarely are they diagnostic of a specific compound.

Other spectroscopic methods are more satisfactory in determining the presence of isolated carbonyl and olefinic bonds. Although isolated double bonds have their maxima around 190 mμ, this is below the satisfactory operating limit of most routine spectrometers. Instrumental features due to energy loss and scattered light, result in inaccuracies below 205 mμ which limit the usefulness of the method for this particular purpose. However cleavage of the olefin to a dicarbonyl compound followed by examination of the class of ketone produced provides a satisfactory method for the determination of olefin type.

2.2. APPLICATIONS OF INFRARED SPECTROSCOPY

Whereas absorption of energy in the ultraviolet region of the spectrum corresponds to electronic transitions, absorption in the infrared region involves changes in molecular vibrations. Of interest to the steroid chemist are those vibrations involving hydroxyl —O—H stretching, carbonyl $>$C$=$O stretching and the olefinic absorptions since these involve the most common functional groups. The typical regions of the spectrum are exemplified by that of dehydroisoandrosterone (Fig. 1).

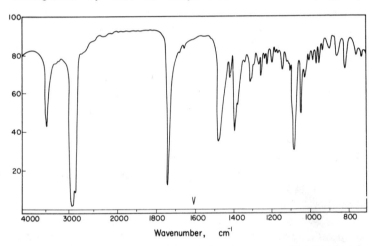

FIG. 1. Infrared spectrum of dehydroisandrosterone as Nujol Mull.

Spectra are determined in a number of ways. The majority of steroids are solids and their spectra are determined as solutions in CS_2, $CHCl_3$ or CCl_4. By choosing solutions of appropriate dilution (0·01 M) interactions between different solute molecules can be minimized. Alternatively spectra may be determined by using a mull of the solid in liquid paraffin (nujol) or hexchlorobutadiene. Another procedure is to take an intimate mixture of the substance and potassium bromide and cast this under pressure in the form of a disc. All these methods utilize 2–3 mg of material although refined techniques using microcells can accommodate smaller samples. The intensity of an infrared band is proportional to the square of the change in dipole moment during the vibration (i.e. useful correlations involve polar functional groups). Since these groups may also be the sites of solvation, care must be taken in extending results from one solvent or phase to another.

The variety of structural possibilities amongst the steroids have led, since the development of recording spectrometers in the late 1940's, to a series of valuable correlations. Indeed if the spectrum does not contain an absorption typical of a certain functional group it almost precludes the presence of that group in the molecule.

Hydroxyl groups

The hydroxyl stretching vibrations which occurs in the range $3450–3650$ cm^{-1} (occasionally as low as 3200 cm^{-1}) forms a valuable diagnostic correlation. The actual position of the absorption is extremely sensitive to the environment of the hydroxyl group particularly to the possibilities of hydrogen bonding. Thus a free non-bonded hydroxyl may absorb between 3650 and 3590 cm^{-1} whilst the hydrogen-bonded absorption occurs at lower frequency (down to 3450 cm^{-1}). Intramolecular bonding may be distinguished from intermolecular hydrogen bonding as the latter is dependent on concentration. Information on the proximity of oxygen functions can be obtained from hydrogen-bonding studies. For example, there is a correlation between the frequency difference of bonded and non-bonded absorption and the length of a hydrogen bond. This feature has been utilized in the study of the stereochemistry of α-glycols as, for example, in the epimeric cholestane-6:7-diols. Transannular hydrogen bonding is frequently encountered and revealed by infrared spectroscopy. For example, cholestan-3α,5β-diol (5) shows absorption at 3620 cm^{-1} whereas cholestan-3α,5α-diol (6) shows two bands at 3620 cm^{-1} and 3521 cm^{-1}. Characteristically the hydrogen-bonded band is a broadened absorption. Carboxylic acids particularly in the solid state, show very marked hydrogen bonding which can produce absorption as low as 2700 cm^{-1}.

Although differences do exist in the C—O stretching region between 1050 and 1200 cm^{-1} to distinguish primary, secondary and tertiary alcohols in different stereochemical environments, nevertheless these correlations are not reliable as they may be confused with other absorptions in this fingerprint region. Furthermore, definitive information on this point can be obtained from n.m.r. spectroscopy.

Carbonyl absorption

The carbonyl group gives rise to absorption in the range 1660–1850 cm.$^{-1}$ In particular the position of absorption is sensitive to ring size and to the presence of conjugated unsaturation. Thus a cyclopentanone absorbs in the range 1735–1750 cm^{-1} whilst a cyclohexanone in the range 1700–1710 cm^{-1} and a cyclohexenone in the range 1670–1690 cm^{-1}. Esters such as acetates absorb at 1735–1745 cm^{-1} whilst a γ-lactone (1760–1780 cm^{-1}) may be distinguished from a δ-lactone (1735–1750 cm^{-1})(see Table 3). A number of other features within the molecule can alter the position of carbonyl absorption. For example, transannular hydrogen bonding between a 5β-

TABLE 3. CARBONYL INFRARED ABSORPTION

	cm^{-1}			cm^{-1}
Ketones		Carboxylic acids		
Acyclic unconj.	1700–1725		Unconj.	1700–1725
Acyclic conj.	1660–1695		Conj.	1680–1715
Cyclic 6-ring unconj.	1700–1720	Esters		
Cyclic 6-ring conj.	1670–1695		Unconj.	1730–1750
Cyclic 5-ring unconj.	1735–1750		Conj.	1715–1730
Cyclic 5-ring conj.	1715–1735	Lactones		
Cyclic 4-ring	1760–1780	δ-Lactones		1735–1750
		γ-Lactones		1755–1780
Aldehydes				
Unconj.	1720–1740	Butenolides		
Conj.	1685–1705			1785–1805

hydroxyl and a 3β-acetoxyl group may alter the acetate absorption. Again a halogen on a α-carbon atom raises the carbonyl absorption by about 20 cm^{-1} provided the carbon-halogen bond is coplanar with carbonyl bond — a feature which was of value in determining the conformation of some ring A 2-bromo-3-keto steroids.

Since carbonyl groups in a number of steroidal positions (e.g. 11) do not readily form derivatives the value of these correlations is immediately apparent. The standard experimental procedure is to determine the spectrum first and then to decide which are the most appropriate derivatives to prepare.

Olefinic absorptions

Non-conjugated olefinic stretching vibrations occur in the range 1620–1680 cm^{-1} whilst a characteristic series of C—H bending frequencies are found in the range 690–995 cm^{-1} the actual position of which is dependent on the substitution pattern of the olefin (see Table 4). The C—H stretching vibration may just be distinguished in the range 3010–3095 as distinct

TABLE 4. OLEFINIC INFRARED ABSORPTION

Type	C—H str.	C=C str.	C—H bending
—CH=CH$_2$	3075–3095 w	1640–1650 m	985–995 s 905–915 s
>C=CH$_2$	3075–3095 w	1650–1660 m	885–895 s
H, H >C=C< (cis)	3010–3030 w	1640–1660	670–730 s
H >C=C< H (trans)	3010–3030	1665–1675	960–980 s
>C=C< H	3010–3040	1665–1675	790–850 s
>C=C<	–	1665–1675	–

from the saturated C—H absorption between 2850 and 3000 cm^{-1}. Conjugated dienes and aromatic compounds show absorption in the range near 1600 cm^{-1} and sometimes also near 1500 cm^{-1}. Whilst a number of absorption bands due to aromatic C—H bending vibrations occur in the range 670–1000 cm^{-1}, these have found little application in steroid chemistry. Although the olefinic C—H out of plane bending frequencies are of considerable diagnostic value, often absorptions due to other modes may appear in the 650–1000 cm^{-1} region. Thus 5α-cholest-1-ene exhibits three appreciable bands in the region 700–750 cm^{-1} at 701, 720 and 746 cm^{-1}.

However, n.m.r. spectroscopy also gives very clear information on the presence of olefinic protons and hence consistent results may also be sought from this method.

Other correlations

The region below 1450 cm^{-1} is often described as the fingerprint region of the spectrum containing many skeletal vibrations. This is of particular value in confirming the identity of two samples. Furthermore, it is often possible to detect minor "extra" bands in this region due to the presence of impurities whose absorption in the main functional group regions may be obscured by other powerful chromophores.

2.3. NUCLEAR MAGNETIC RESONANCE SPECTROSCOPY

Three valuable classes of information can be obtained from the nuclear magnetic resonance spectrum of a compound. The position of a proton resonance gives a clear indication of its chemical environment whilst the integral corresponds to the relative number of protons contributing to a given resonance. From the multiplicity of a resonance it is possible to gain information about the number and steric relationship of neighbouring protons. In favourable circumstances this feature can be confirmed by double-irradiation experiments. Useful spectra may be obtained with 15–25 mg steroid dissolved in deuterochloroform (0·4 ml) whilst in exceptional cases much smaller amounts can be studied by using a computer to sum the result of many sweeps (C.A.T. = computer of average transients). The major useful regions of the spectrum are summarized in Fig. 2. A typical 100 Mc spectrum, that of dehydroisoandrosterone, is illustrated in Fig. 3. Although routine n.m.r. spectroscopy of steroids is a comparatively recent innovation, the numerous structural correlations that have been made clearly demonstrate the value of the technique. Useful ultraviolet

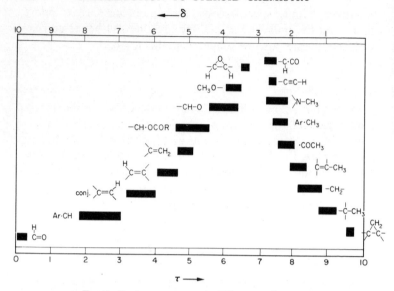

FIG. 2. Proton resonances in different environments.

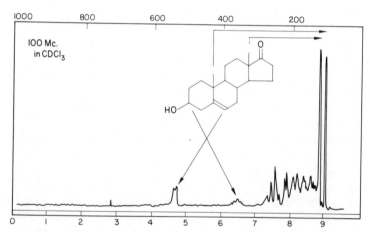

FIG. 3. Nuclear magnetic resonance spectrum of dehydroisoandrosterone.

spectroscopy is restricted to conjugated chromophores whilst infrared spectroscopy gives invaluable information on functional groups. The information obtained from n.m.r. spectroscopy complements this in that it is concerned with the differing environment of protons — of which the average steroid contains between forty and fifty.

The most distinctive features of many steroid spectra are the sharp three-proton singlets assigned to the angular methyl resonances at C-18 and C-19. These have been distinguished and in the saturated hydrocarbon 5α-androstane appear at $\tau 9 \cdot 308$ and $\tau 9 \cdot 208$, respectively. Transannular interactions with hydroxyl, ketonic olefinic and epoxide functions serve to modify these positions. Within certain limits these effects are approximately additive and an extensive tabulation of chemical shifts due to substituents in various locations has been compiled. In polyfunctional steroids some caution has to be exercized as interaction between two functional groups will obviously affect the magnetic susceptibility and hence their influence on the angular group. In particular $\alpha\beta$-unsaturated ketones and allylic alcohols have to be considered as entities. Further deviations from these positions arise due to skeletal deformations such as alteration in the conformation of a ring. Dipole–dipole interactions may cause a functional group to take up an unusual conformation and this in turn, will be reflected in its effect on the field experienced by an angular group. In the extreme case of the inversion of ring A from a chair to a boat form, this can cause the angular C-19 methyl group to move from the deshielding region of a 3-carbonyl group into the shielding cone.

Methyl groups attached to double bonds appear at lower field and as they are of less common occurrence in steroid work, they may be easily recognized. Many methyl ketones and acetates occur and these may be clearly recognized by resonances in range $\tau 7 \cdot 9 – 8 \cdot 1$. In general protons attached to carbon bearing a singly bonded oxygen appear in the range $\tau 5 \cdot 0 – 6 \cdot 7$. The position and shape of the proton resonance is dependent not only on its axial or equatorial nature but also on the number and orientation of the neighbouring protons. As a general rule axial ring protons [equatorial C—O] resonate at a higher field than their epimeric counterparts. Furthermore, the parent alcohol will appear at higher field ($\tau 5 \cdot 5 - 6 \cdot 5$) than the corresponding acetate ($\tau 4 \cdot 6 - 5 \cdot 6$). Methyl esters appear as a sharp singlet near $\tau 6 \cdot 3$ whilst steroidal epoxide protons occur in the range $\tau 6 \cdot 5 - 7 \cdot 2$. The hydroxyl proton resonance is markedly affected by hydrogen bonding and does not have a characteristic position in the spectrum. It may be eliminated by shaking with deuterium oxide or trifluoroacetic acid. However, the rate of proton exchange which normally prevents it showing coupling through oxygen to the carbon–hydrogen protons is sufficiently reduced in dimethylsulphoxide solution to permit the observation of hydroxyl proton splitting. Hence in this solvent primary, secondary and tertiary alcohols may give triplets, doublets and singlets, respectively. Normally they are, of course, distinguished by the integral.

Considerable structural information has been obtained with steroidal acetates and α-acetoxy ketones by a study of the coupling constants. The relationship between the vicinal coupling constant and the dihedral angle has been summarized in terms of the Karplus equation, $J = A \cos^2\phi - B$, where A and B are constants. A may lie between $8 \cdot 5$ and 10 for $0° \leqslant \phi \leqslant 90°$ and between $9 \cdot 5$ and 10 for $90° \leqslant \phi \leqslant 180°$, whilst B is approximately $0 \cdot 28$. The magnitude of A would appear to vary with the nature of the substituents and hence only approximate dihedral angles can be calculated. However, by utilizing epimeric pairs of compounds it is possible to distinguish between axial and equatorial isomers and between chair and boat forms.

The variation of coupling constant with dihedral angle is shown in Fig. 4. This is based on the Williamson and Johnson modification of the Karplus equation. In the steroid field measurements of this kind have been applied to the conformations of ring A utilizing 2α- and β-acetoxy-3-ketones.

The coupling of one proton to an adjacent proton may be

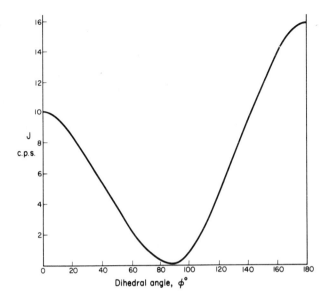

Fɪɢ. 4. Variation of coupling constant with dihedral angle.

confirmed by the application of double resonance or spin-decoupling. This experiment is applicable in cases where the proton resonances are well separated. One resonance is strongly irradiated and the protons thus transferred to one spin-state. This removes the coupling to the second proton which is then scanned. There are a number of important applications of spin

TABLE 5. VARIATION OF COUPLING
CONSTANT WITH DIHEDRAL ANGLE

		Calc.	Obs.
$\phi_{a.a}$	180°	9–16	8–14
$\phi_{a.e}$	60°	1·8–2·5	1–7
$\phi_{e.e}$	60°	1·8–2·5	1–7

decoupling. Firstly, this confirms and simplifies coupling patterns. Secondly, it may enable the determination of the position of a resonance which is itself completely obscured by other resonances but which is coupled to a second proton with an observable pattern. Thirdly, it becomes possible to demonstrate couplings which may not immediately be obvious. Thus there are some examples of long-range coupling in the steroids which have been revealed in this manner.

The olefinic region ($\tau 3 \cdot 5 - 5 \cdot 0$) of the n.m.r. spectrum can be useful in defining the double-bond type. The relative number of protons obtained by the integral together with their multiplicity can give a strong indication of the substitution pattern. Various examples are shown in Fig. 5.

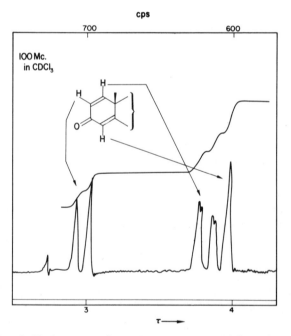

FIG. 5. Nuclear magnetic resonance spectrum (olefin region) of cholesta-1,4-diene-3-one.

Allylic coupling can lead to definite assignments of the olefinic resonances. Hence taken in conjunction with other physical methods, considerable structural information is available on double-bond types.

For many purposes spectra are determined in deuterochloroform solution. However, information can be obtained by comparing spectra obtained in different solvents. For example, by using an aromatic solvent such as pyridine or benzene which selectively solvates functions such as hydroxyls and ketones, the anisotropic effect of the solvent ring current may differentially shift the resonance of various solute protons. In this manner overlapping multiplets can be clarified. Furthermore, a $1:3$ chemical interaction between, for example, a hydroxyl and methyl group can be demonstrated (e.g. 6β-hydroxy steroids).

2.4. APPLICATION OF MASS SPECTROMETRY

The advent of high resolution mass spectrometers capable of handling compounds with a low volatility and a molecular weight of up to 1000, has placed this method within the range of the steroid chemist. As a consequence over the last few years there have been an increasing number of papers devoted to the mass spectrometry of steroids. From these a number of applications are apparent. Firstly, the method is of primary importance in determining very accurate molecular weights and hence the elemental composition of unknown steroids. Irrespective of any information derived from the fragmentation pattern, the recognition of the molecular ion is of considerable value. For example, analytical data had not distinguished between $C_{32}H_{48}O_8$ and $C_{33}H_{50}O_8$ formulations for the steroidal antibiotic cephalosporin P. The mass spectrum gave an unequivocal answer.

The steroid skeleton, unlike certain other groups of natural product, does not possess any specific bond which undergoes fission in the mass spectrometer. Hence the fragmentation is susceptible to the directing influence of certain substituents.

Unfortunately the two commonest functional groups, the hydroxyl and carbonyl groups, do not appear to cause a steroid to fragment in any general manner and hence it is difficult at present to predict the fragmentation pattern of a polysubstituted steroid. However, sufficient model compounds have been studied for it to be possible, once a hydroxy or keto-steroid has been place in a class, to decide whether the fragmentation pattern is consistent with, for example, the location of a carbonyl group at C-7 or C-17.

The fragmentation patterns of carbonyl compounds reveal a number of rearrangement processes which have been studied by deuterium exchange. One of the most common of these is the cleavage of a β-bond with the transfer of a γ-hydrogen atom to the carbonyl group (7). Rearrangements of this kind, exemplified by the fragmentation of a 16-ketone (8), are dependent upon conformation. Indeed although the carbonyl group may not be strongly directing in steroid fragmentation, differences between two closely related compounds, such as the intensity of a M-70 peak corresponding to the loss of ring A in 5α- and 5β-cholestan-3-one, may be evident from the mass spectrum.

7

8

9

Two groups, the ethylene ketal and dimethylamino functions, have been shown to direct fragmentation in a fairly predictable manner. The two adjacent oxygen atoms of the ketal can stabilize the positive charge of an ion (9) after homolytic fission of the carbon–carbon bond adjacent to the functional group. Thus breakdown of ring A in a 3-ethylene ketal to give *inter alia* a fragment m/e 99 [(10)–(11)] has been substantiated by deuterium labelling.

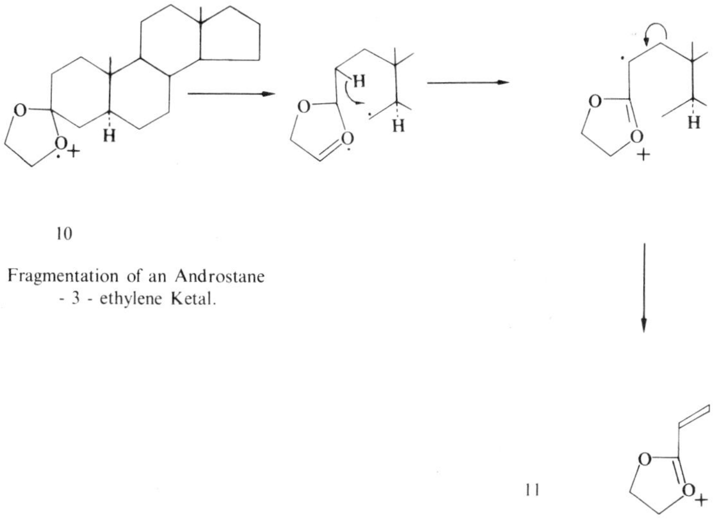

10

Fragmentation of an Androstane
    - 3 - ethylene Ketal.

11

m/e 99

In the case of the oestrogenic hormones in which ring A is aromatic, the molecular-ion forms a strong peak. Indeed this is sufficiently strong for mass spectrometry to be of possible value in association with vapour phase chromatography in the biochemical analysis of oestrogenic hormones. The fragmentation of the oestrogens is initiated by benzylic cleavage, for example in the formation of m/e 160 in the breakdown of oestrone methyl ether [(12)–(13)].

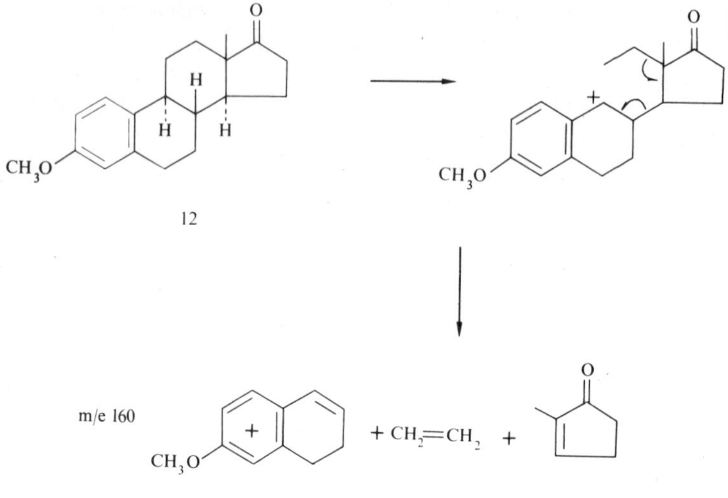

12

m/e 160

13

A number of thermal eliminations, such as dehydration and the 1:2-elimination of acetic acid, can occur in the mass spectrometer. The presence of the relevant M-18 and M-60 peaks can be of value in the identification of these groups. Hence taken in conjunction with other physical methods, mass spectrometry can aid the steroid chemist. One of its particular virtues is the small amount of material required for each determination.

2.5. OPTICAL ROTATION

The use of optical rotation in the assignment of structure to steroids and their derivatives has been considerable. The basis of the method is that provided the centres of asymmetry are sufficiently far apart, then their contributions to the overall molecular rotations are independent and separable. In this analysis it is fortunate that the steroid molecule is relatively flat and that in many compounds the functional groups are well-separated. Features such as the introduction of bulky axial substituents, which may lead to skeletal deformations and the possibility of interactions such as hydrogen-bonding between substituents, have provided limitations to the application of the method. The Method of Molecular Rotation Differences assumes that the molecular rotation of a steroid may be made up of the rotation due to the fundamental carbon skeleton (androstane, cholestane, pregnane series) to which the rotation contribution of the functional groups (Δ-values) are added. The Δ-values are characteristic of the position and orientation of the substituents and are within limits, independent of each other.

An extension of the method utilizes the difference in molecular rotation between the acetate, benzoate or ketone and the corresponding secondary alcohol. These are known as Δ_1, Δ_2 and Δ_3 values respectively. Some examples for the cholestan-3-ols are shown in Table 6. However, the introduction of olefin

TABLE 6

	Δ_1	Δ_2	Δ_3
5α-cholestan-3β-ol	-29	$+5$	$+73$
5α-cholestan-3α-ol	$+17$	$+17$	$+66$
Δ^5-cholestene-3β-ol	-34	$+80$	$+124$

and carbonyl as a neighbour can influence the contribution to the molecular rotation by a group. For example, 3-hydroxy steroidal-5-enes and -6-ketones show a marked divergence from the calculated Δ_3-values. With the advent of other spectroscopic and more refined optical methods the application of this technique has lessened in recent years. Nevertheless, it still remains a useful guide to the stereochemistry of steroids.

2.6. OPTICAL ROTATORY DISPERSION AND CIRCULAR DICHROISM

The method of molecular rotation differences utilizes one wavelength only, normally the sodium D line (589 mμ). However, the variation of optical rotation with wavelength (optical rotatory dispersion) has led to some valuable correlations. Plane-polarized light comprises two equal and opposite circular vectors. A difference in the rate of transmission of one of these leads to a rotation of the plane polarization when the vectors are recombined. If unequal absorption of the left- and right-handed vectors occurs then the resultant beam of light is elliptically polarized. The variation of this latter feature with wavelength in the region of an optically active chromophore

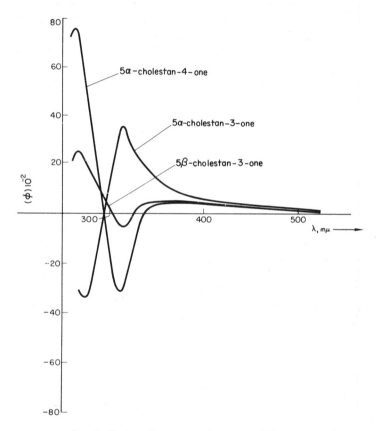

FIG. 6. Cotton-effect curves of some steroid ketones.

is known as circular dichroism and leads to a Cotton effect in the optical rotatory dispersion curve. The development of spectropolarimeters capable of operating in the ultraviolet region has led to an extensive application of this method in steroid chemistry.

The first chromophore to be examined in detail was the carbonyl group. Some typical examples of steroidal curves are shown.

It can be seen that the curves show a peak and trough known as the Cotton effect in the region of the $n-\pi^*$ transition of the carbonyl group. The sign and shape of this effect is dependent on the environment of the chromophore. An application, namely that of locating a carbonyl group on the steroid, is immediately obvious. By studying the influence of substituents, particularly α-haloketones, a rule for predicting the sign of Cotton effect has been developed.

This rule, known as the Octant Rule, has some theoretical justification. The ring containing the carbonyl group is viewed as shown in Fig. 7 and then three planes at right angles are drawn through the carbonyl group to produce eight octants.

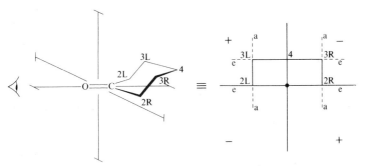

Fig. 7. Octant rule and projection for a ketone.

The contribution of a substituent to the sign of the Cotton effect depends on its position in these octants. Taking the rear four octants these are summarized in Fig. 7. The application of the rule can be exemplified by considering cholestan-4-one (Fig. 8), for which a negative Cotton effect is predicted. The application of optical rotatory dispersion to stereochemical problems in the steroid field can be exemplified in a number of ways. A special case of the Octant Rule is the axial haloketone

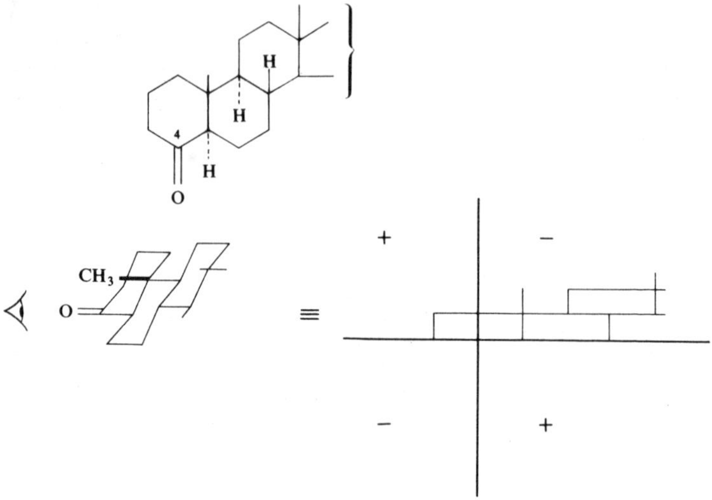

FIG. 8. Octant projection for a 4-ketone.

rule. The introduction of an axial chlorine or bromine next to the keto group of a cyclohexanone affects the sign of the Cotton effect and hence the orientation and position of substitution becomes apparent. For example, bromination of 2α-methyl-cholestan-3-one gave a 2-bromo derivative possessing a negative Cotton effect and an axially oriented halogen. This result can only be accommodated by a 2α-bromo-2β-methyl structure in which ring A adopts a boat conformation. The assignment of configuration at C-5 to the reduction products of Δ^4-cholesten-3-ones has presented structural problems. However, there is a marked difference between the rotatory dispersion curves of 3-keto steroids epimeric at C-5, a feature which was utilized in assigning the stereochemistry of the reduction products of 19-nortestosterone. In other series such as the tetracyclic diterpenoids where antipodal A/B fusions occur, the optical rotatory dispersion curves are important in assigning the optical series.

Indeed the application of optical rotatory dispersion to more highly substituted steroidal systems has revealed a number of examples in which rings adopt boat and twist conformations. Thus 2β-acetoxycholestan-3-one shows a different amplitude from the parent ketone suggesting that it has adopted a modified ring A conformation in order to relieve the strong $1:3$ diaxial interaction between the 2β-acetoxy and 10β-methyl groups. Similarly the method can reveal long-range skeletal distortions arising through conformational transmission.

For instrumental reasons the amplitude of the Cotton effect is less accurately measured. However, by adding acid to methanol solutions of steroidal ketones it is possible to follow the formation of methoxy-ketal derivatives.

A number of other chromophores, such as acetates, lactones and nitro-compounds, have been studied. Since optical rotation and circular dichroism are sensitive to conformational features which in turn vary with temperature a number of low-temperature studies have been conducted with the aim of studying conformationally mobile systems.

The various physical methods that are available to the steroid chemist are complementary in the information that can be obtained from them. On the whole the results are those derived from a series of empirical correlations with model compounds. It should therefore be evident that deductions should be made from a several methods rather than too great a reliance placed on any one.

READING REFERENCES

Textbooks

U.V.   A. I. SCOTT, *Interpretation of the Ultraviolet Spectra of Natural Products.*

I.R.   L. J. Bellamy, *The Infra-red Spectra of Complex Molecules*.
             K. Nakanishi, *Infrared Absorption Spectroscopy*.
             A. D. Cross, *Practical Infrared Spectroscopy*.
N.M.R.   L. M. Jackmann, *Applications of N.M.R. Spectroscopy in Organic Chemistry*.
             N. S. Bhacca and D. H. Williams, *Applications of N.M.R. Spectroscopy in Organic Chemistry*.
Mass Spectra H. Budzikiewicz, C. Djerassi and D. H. Williams, *Interpretation of Mass Spectra of Organic Compounds*.
O.R.D./C.D. C. Djerassi, *Optical Rotatory Dispersion*.
             P. Crabbé, *Optical Rotatory Dispersion and Circular Dichroism*.

Review articles

U.V.   L. Dorfmann, *Chem. Rev.* **53**, 47 (1953).
I.R.   A. R. H. Cole, *Fortschr. Chem. Org. Naturstoffe* **13**, 1 (1956).
N.M.R.   R. F. Zurcher, *Helv. Chim. Acta* **46**, 2054 (1963).
             A. I. Cohen and S. Rock, *Steroids* **3**, 243 (1964).
O.R.D./C.D. W. Klyne, *Advances in Organic Chemistry,* Vol. 1, p. 239, Interscience, New York, 1960.
             C. Djerassi, *Proc. Chem. Soc.* 314 (1964).
             W. Klyne, *Stereochemical Correlations,* R.I.C. Lecture Series, No. 4 (1962).

CHAPTER 3

The Conformational Analysis of Steroid Reactions

THE methods of conformational analysis have been widely employed in elucidating the stereochemical consequences of steroid reactions. In the absence of distorting effects such as hydrogen-bonding and electrostatic interactions, the most stable conformation of a molecule is the one in which non-bonded interactions are minimized. When this is applied to the boat (1) and chair (2) conformations of a cyclohexane ring it is evident that the chair form, in which all the C—H bonds on adjacent carbon atoms are staggered, will be the more stable.

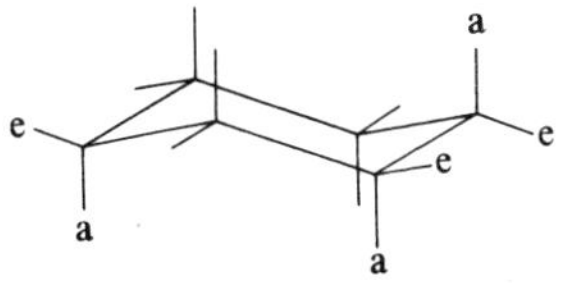

1

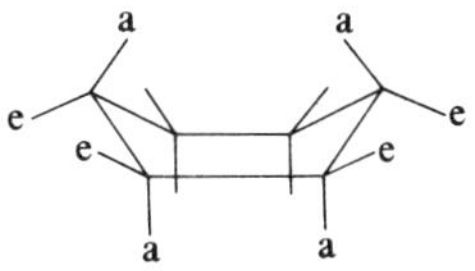

2

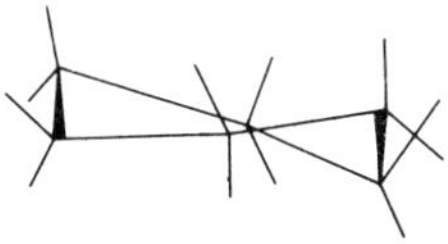

3

A twist form (3) which may be regarded as an intermediate boat form, permits the relief of strong 1:4 interactions present in the complete boat form. It seems likely that some steroid ring systems take up this conformation. When a substituent occupies the axial conformation on a chair cyclohexane ring it is usually subjected to greater non-bonded interactions (1:3 interactions) than when it is in the equatorial conformation. Hence the stable conformation of a mobile substituted cyclohexane ring is that in which the greatest number of substituents occupy equatorial positions.

The polycyclic steroid framework imposes a rigidity on the component cyclohexane rings. Both the 5α-cholestane and 5β-cholestane (coprostane) series can attain the all-chair forms

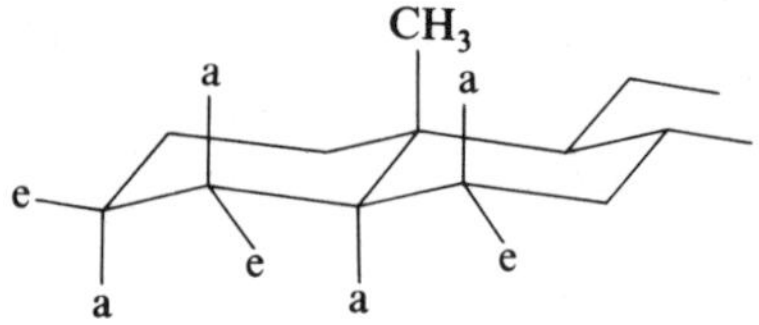

4

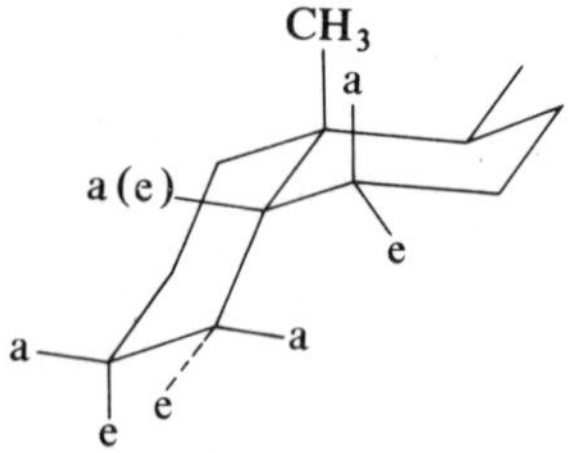

5

—a feature confirmed in the solid state by X-ray analysis. There is then a definite relationship between configuration and conformation. These relationships are shown in (4) and (5). The difference between the *cis* and *trans* fused A/B systems is then reflected in the different conformations of α and β substituents on ring A. Furthermore, it is apparent that the interactions of the 2 and 4 positions with ring B contribute to diminish the stability of the *cis* fused 5β-cholestane (coprostane) system relative to the *trans* fused 5α-cholestane.

However, in unusual circumstances boat forms may occur. For example, potentially equatorial α-bromoketones tend to distort away from the chain form to relieve the repulsion between the equatorial C-Br and the adjacent carbonyl dipoles. In extreme cases complete inversion to the conformer with an axial bromine atom may happen. This has formed the subject of study with 2α-bromo-3-keto cholestane and its relatives which possess a flexible ring A.

The application of detailed physical measurements to the determination of the conformation of a steroid has been outlined in Chapter 2. It is one of the features of the application of conformational analysis to steroid reactions that information on the ground state conformation of a molecule obtained from physical measurements and by inspection of molecule models, may in most circumstances be directly extended to the transition state of a reacting molecule. In doing this care must be taken to distinguish between those features which affect the transition states of two competing reactions and lead to kinetic control of the products and those features which contribute to the relative stability of two possible end products—in an equilibrating process the features which lead to thermodynamic control of the products.

Although these two features are interrelated, for the purposes of this discussion we will treat them separately and describe firstly some examples of the effect of conformation on the rates of reaction and then secondly its effect on the products of reaction.

3.1. EFFECT OF CONFORMATION ON RATES OF REACTIONS

(a) *Rates of esterification and hydrolysis*

In the formation and hydrolysis of esters we are concerned with the relative ease of attack of axial and equitorial centres. In this context an equatorial centre is more readily attacked than its axial epimer. This may be exempled in the difference in the rate of hydrolysis of acetates at various centres. This is shown in formula (6) which indicates the epimer that is more rapidly hydrolysed.

It has been found that in some circumstances the mono acetates of 1:3-diaxial diols are hydrolysed much faster than is usual for axial acetates. The interactions leading to

this phenomenon are illustrated in the hydrolysis of 3α-acetoxy-5α-hydroxycholestane (7). In the diaxial (3α,5α- and 3β,5β-isomers) the hydroxyl group is suitably situated for hydrogen-bonding to the ester and so can facilitate its hydrolysis. This type of transannular neighbouring group participation can contribute to a variety of steroidal reactions.

The solvolysis of a leaving group may involve nucleophilic substitution at a cyclic carbon atom. In bimolecular solvolysis, this involves the approach of the reagent from the opposite side of the carbon atom. For an equatorial substituent approach is hindered by other axial substituents on the ring system. On the other hand, the approach of a nucleophile to the rear of an axial substituent involves interaction only with the adjacent groups. For this reason axial groups such as an 11β-bromo group are solvolysed more rapidly than the corresponding equatorial epimer by hydroxide ion. Since O-alkyl solvolysis proceeds with inversion it can provide a way of making some less readily available steroids. Thus the toluene-*p*-sulphonate of 3β-hydroxy-5α-cholestane on solvolysis with potassium acetate in acetic acid gives *inter alia* 3α-hydroxy-5α-cholestane. Transannular reactions are found in the solvolysis of 5α-hydroxy-3β-tosyloxycholestane (8) in which the nucleophile is the anion derived from the 5α-hydroxyl group. The second product (9) in which ring A has been cleaved arises from a fragmentation reaction.

In S$_N$1 substitution reactions such as the acetolysis of cholestanyl tosylates the rate of the reaction has been correlated with relief of steric compression associated with the departure of the leaving group. A similar feature must also affect the rate of E.1 elimination in which the formation of a carbonium ion plays an important part.

When the conformational differences between the reactivity of alcohols is taken to its extreme a number of selective reactions are observed. For example, selective hydrolysis of the diacetate of 3β,6β-dihydroxy-5α-cholestane leads to the 6-monoacetate. The axial 6-acetate is hindered by a 1:3 diaxial interaction with the angular methyl group and on the other hand by two 1:3 interactions with hydrogen. Similarly it is difficult to acetylate the 11β-hydroxyl group, because of the two strong 1:3 diaxial interactions. Cholic acid shows a marked distinction in reactivity between the 3α-, 7α- and 12α-hydroxyls.

For example treatment of methyl cholate with excess ethyl-chlorocarbonate yields methyl cholate 3-cathylate in high yield. Acetylation on the other hand yields mainly the 3,7-diacetate leaving the 12-position unattacked.

(b) *Oxidation of alcohols*

The rate of oxidation of alcohols to their corresponding ketones is susceptible to conformational factors. Oxidation with chromic acid requires the formation of a chromate ester and the subsequent fission of the C—H bond. It is this latter stage which represents in the majority of cases the rate-determining step. In an equatorial alcohol the C—H bond has the less accessible axial conformation. Hence an equatorial alcohol is oxidized slower than its axial epimer. Different centres in the steroid nucleus are oxidized at differing rates (see Table 1) and it appears that the reaction rate is dependent on the decrease in steric interactions on the formation of the trigonal centre of the carbonyl group.

TABLE 1. RELATIVE RATES OF OXIDATION OF SOME
STEROIDAL ALCOHOLS WITH CHROMIUM TRIOXIDE
(5α-cholestan-3β-ol = 1)

Axial alcohol		Equatorial alcohol	
5α-cholestan-1α-ol	13·0	5α-cholestan-1β-ol	9·7
5α-cholestan-2β-ol	20·0	5α-cholestan-2α-ol	1·3
5α-cholestan-3α-ol	3·0	5α-cholestan-3β-ol	1·0
5α-cholestan-4β-ol	35·0	5α-cholestan-4α-ol	2·0
5α-cholestan-6β-ol	36	5α-cholestan-6α-ol	2·0
5α-cholestan-7α-ol	12·3	5α-cholestan-7β-ol	3·3

The oxidation of vicinal diols by sodium periodate and lead tetraacetate has been studied in rings A and B of the steroids. As would be expected there are differences in rate between epimers. The energy required to bring two adjacent equatorial bonds on a cyclohexane ring into the same plane is greater than that which is used to make adjacent axial and equatorial bonds coplanar. In the case of the former this produces angle strain whilst the latter involves the formation of a half boat form. The results of kinetic studies on the oxidation of the isomeric $3\beta,6,7$-trihydroxy-5α-cholestane glycols exemplify this. The diaxial $6\beta,7\alpha$-isomer is unattacked whilst the diequatorial $6\alpha,7\beta$-isomer reacts less rapidly than the two axialequatorial glycols.

3.2. EFFECT OF CONFORMATION ON THE PRODUCTS OF A REACTION

The preceding discussion has been devoted to reaction rates. However, for many reactions the transition state imposes certain constraints on the possible products which may be influenced by the stereochemical environment of the reacting centre.

(a) *Addition reactions*

The addition reactions of steroidal olefins which proceed through cyclic "onium" ions such as the bromonium ion yield *trans* diaxial products. In this way the four participating centres are most nearly coplanar in the transition state. For example, the addition of bromine to cholesteryl acetate yields the $5\alpha,6\beta$-dibromide whilst the addition to 5α-cholest-2-ene affords $2\beta,3\alpha$-dibromo-5α-cholestane as the main product. In the latter case this presumably proceeds through the $2\alpha,3\alpha$-bromonium ion, initial attack having been directed to the "α" face of the molecule by the angular methyl group. Similarly the addition of hypobromous acid to 5α-cholest-2-ene affords mainly the diaxial 3α-bromo-2β-hydroxy-5α-cholestane.

The geometrical preference of four coplanar reaction centres dominates both the formation of epoxide rings from halo-hydrins and the hydrolysis of epoxides. This may also be exemplified from the reactions of ring A. Thus the diaxial bromohydrins 3α-bromo-2β-hydroxy-5α-cholestane and 2β-bromo-3α-hydroxy-5α-cholestane, rapidly undergo epoxide formation. On the other hand, the diequatorial 2α-bromo-3β-hydroxy-5α-cholestane reacts very slowly. Hydrolysis of cholestane-2α-epoxide gives the diaxial $2\beta,3\alpha$-bromohydrin rather than the alternative *trans* diequatorial $3\beta,2\alpha$-bromohydrin.

Another stereochemical feature dominates the *cis* addition to double bonds in the steroid framework. Bulky reagents which add in this fashion attack from the less-hindered face of the molecule. The axial β-oriented C-18 and C-19 methyl groups hinder the approach of reagents to the β-face of 5α-steroids leading to the "Rule of α attack". Hydroxylations with potassium permanganate and osmium tetroxide, epoxidation with peracids, and hydroboration reactions take place from the "α" face of the molecule. This is demonstrated in the reactions of the $5:6$ double bond of cholesterol. Thus oxidation of cholesterol with osmium tetroxide gives the $3\beta,5\alpha,$ 6α-triol whilst expoxidation with perbenzoic acid forms mainly the "α" epoxide. The latter is hydrolysed to the diaxial $3\beta,5\alpha,6\beta$-triol. This same triol is produced by the addition of performic acid and hydrolysis of the intermediate 3,6-diformate. Hydroboration of cholesterol acetate produces the 6α-alcohol. Catalytic hydrogenation of cholesterol yields 5α-cholestan-3β-ol with the 5α addition of hydrogen. On the other hand, catalytic reduction of Δ^4-cholestene gives coprostane (with a 5β addition of hydrogen).

(b) *Reduction of ketones*

The reduction of steroidal ketones exemplifies a number of stereochemical features that may influence reactions. In this respect reducing agents may be divided into a number of classes. These include the hydride reagents, the hydride-transfer agents, the dissolving-metal reagents and the catalytic methods. The major feature that affects the outcome of reduction with the hydride reagents is the steric hindrance to the pathway taken by the attacking hydride ion. In particular approach to the developing transition state is likely to take place from the less-hindered face of the molecule (steric approach control). In a case in which the reagent can approach either face of an unhindered ketone in the developing transition state the possibility of generating a more stable equatorial alcohol ("product development control") then influences the course of the reduction. Thus reduction of the relatively unhindered 5α-cholestan-3-one with lithium aluminium hydride affords the equatorial alcohol 5α-cholestan-3β-ol in 90% yield. On the other hand, reduction of the hindered 5α-cholestan-6-one produces the axial alcohol, 5α-cholestan-6β-ol. These results have been summarized in the statement "reduction of unhindered ketones with sodium borohydride or lithium aluminium hydride tends to give the equatorial alcohol while with the hindered ketones the axial epimer is obtained". The hydride-transfer agents such as the Meerwein–Poondorf reagent require the formation of a bulky complex intermediate. Not only are these reagents likely to give a high proportion of equatorial alcohol but also they can act in a selective manner leaving hindered ketones as at position 11, unattacked. It is possible that this feature of "product development control" is present in the reductions with lithium tri-tertiary-butoxy-aluminium hydride and occasionally with sodium borohydride. Reduction with a dissolving metal reagent such as sodium dissolving in alcohol or lithium in liquid ammonia involves the initial transfer of electrons to the carbonyl group followed by protonation. The electron transfer stage in which the oxygen of the carbonyl groups is free in the transition state to take up the more stable conformation produces the less-hindered — usually equatorial — alcohol. The formation of a carbanion in this process resembles the inter-mediate required in the equilibration of axial and equatorial alcohols under strongly basic conditions (e.g. in the presence of sodium amyloxide). Thus reduction of cholestan-6-one with sodium and ethanol affords the equatorial cholestan-6α-ol. When this process is applied to the reduction of αβ-unsaturated ketones such as cholest-4-en-3-one, the product possesses the more stable *trans* A/B fusion of cholestanone. However, zinc/acetic acid reduction of cholest-4-en-3,6-dione has been observed to give the *cis* A/B fused 5β-cholestan-3,6-dione.

Catalytic reduction is a case in which the ease of approach of the carbonyl group to the activated catalyst surface determines the outcome of the *cis* addition of hydrogen. For this reason in many cases the reduction product can contain a high proportion of the axial alcohol as in rapid catalytic reduction (i.e. under acidic conditions in which there is less chance of any carbanion equilibrium to occur) with a platinum catalyst in acetic acid containing perchloric acid. Catalytic hydrogenation of cholestan-6-one yields the axial alcohol 5α-cholestan-6β-ol.

(c) *Elimination reactions*

The elimination reactions of steroids in many cases accompany and compete with substitution reactions. Bimolecular elimination reactions are facilitated in those instances in which there is a trans diaxial relationship between the participating groups, i.e. a relationship producing a coplanar transition state. Thus cholesterol-5α,6β-dibromide is readily debrominated by iodine whilst the diequatorial isomer — the 5β,6α-dibromide — reacts slowly. This feature can control the double-bond isomer obtained from an elimination reaction. For example, treatment of 3β-methyl-5α-cholestan-3α-ol with phosphorus oxychloride in pyridine results in the formation of 3-methyl-5α-cholest-2-ene whilst the 3β-alcohol which can only achieve a *trans* diaxial relationship with a hydrogen atom of the methyl group, yields the exocyclic olefin. Another more subtle example comes from the elimination reaction of the pregnane 20α-and 20β-tosylates (10) and (11) which yield the isomeric olefins (12) and (13). Elimination takes place from the rotamer in which there is a *trans* diaxial relationship between the leaving group and the 17α-hydrogen atom.

The Hofmann elimination of 4-aza-steroids provides an interesting example of the consequences of this relationship. In the coprostane series diaxial eliminations of (14) affords the olefin (15). However, in the 5α series (16) no axial relationship of this type exists and elimination takes place to form (17) by attack at an equatorial proton.

Olefin formation frequently occurs in the reactions of toluene-*p*-sulphonates. Thus chromatography of the toluene-*p*-sulphonate of 5α-cholestan-3β-ol on alkaline alumina forms a useful preparative method of cholest-2-ene. It is interesting in this respect to note that ionic elimination of a 7β-tosylate on alumina yields cholest-7-ene. On the other hand, pyrolysis of the 7α-benzoate which proceeds through *cis*-elimination by a cyclic mechanism affords cholest-6-ene—there is no 8α-hydrogen atom.

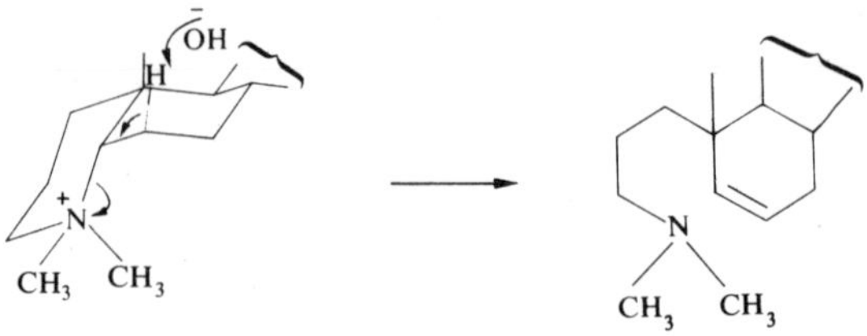

14   15

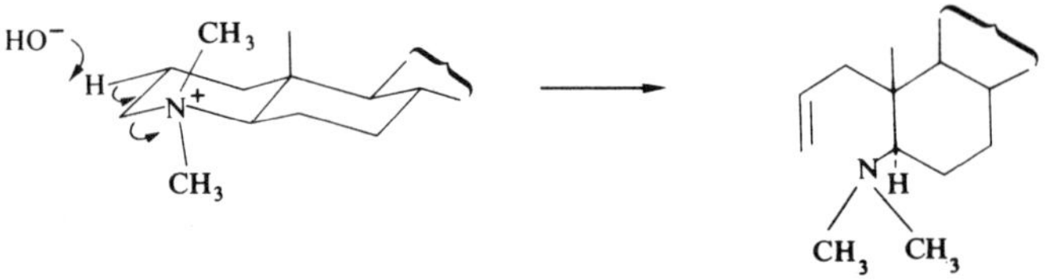

16   17

(d) *Substitution reactions*

The stereochemistry of substitution reactions in the steroids
has been examined in great detail. The replacement of hydroxyl by halogen in particular has been the subject of study.
At C-3 S_N2 nucleophilic substitution proceeds with inversion.
For example 5α-cholestan-3β-ol on treatment with phosphorus
pentachloride affords 5α-cholestan-3α-chloride. On the other
hand, reaction with thionyl chloride which proceeds by the $S_N i$
mechanism yields 5α-cholestan-3β-chloride with retention of
configuration. The influence of environment can be clearly
seen by comparing the result with reaction at C-6. Thus reaction of cholestan-6α-ol with both phosphorus pentachloride
and thionyl chloride proceeds with retention to give 5α-
cholestan-6α-chloride both reactions proceeding by the
$S_N i$ mechanism. In this case the angular methyl group at
C-10 suppresses the S_N2 mechanism by sterically blocking
the incoming group. Treatment of cholestan-6β-ol with these
reagents gives mainly the products of elimination.

Solvolysis of both 3α- and 3β-toluene-*p*-sulphonates and the halides yields the products of inversion and elimination. Thus methanolysis of the 3α-toluene-*p*-sulphonate gives a low yield of the 3β-methyl ether and a larger amount of cholest-2-ene. On the other hand, acetolysis of the alkyl chlorides gives together with the products of inversion and elimination some products of retention possibly through the intervention of an S_N1 component.

The unimolecular solvolysis of the unsaturated cholesterol 3β-toluene-*p*-sulphonate proceeds in a different manner through the intervention of a homoallylic cation to give the characteristic "*i*-steroid" rearrangement products (e.g. 18). The results of this and the solvolysis of the 4:4-dimethyl steroids which result in rearrangement, will be discussed in the next chapter.

18

Deamination reactions of amino-steroids clearly reflect the intervention of a unimolecular mechanism. In general deamination proceeds with retention of configuration. The nitrous acid deamination of the equatorial 2,3,4,6 and 7-aminocholestanes gives the appropriate equatorial alcohol in high yield whilst the axial amines react again with retention, to give a lower yield of the axial alcohol accompanied by the products of elimination.

(e) *Bromination of ketones*

The results of bromination of a number of steroidal ketones have been studied. Initially it was proposed that when a cyclohexanone was brominated under conditions of kinetic control, the major product has the bromine atom in the axial conformation. This generalization is rationalized by assuming that the bromine atom attacks the enol in the direction best suited for maximum overlap with enolate π-orbital. However, more recent studies have been concerned with the reconciliation of this hypothesis with the stereochemical environment of the enolate.

Two features have to be considered. Firstly the direction of enolization of the ketone which controls the site of bromination, and secondly the direction of addition to the enolate which controls the stereochemistry. Subsequently the system may deform to take up a boat conformation to relieve interaction. Thermodynamic control may then occur and produce a more stable (equatorial) isomer. Thus 5α-cholestan-2-one forms a Δ^2-enol-acetate. Axial bromination of the ketone or the enol-acetate affords 3α-bromo-5α-cholestan-2-one.

Perpendicular attack on half chair enolate (19) can occur from two sides which may be distinguished. Attack from the same side as the adjacent pseudo-axial bond known as parallel attack, leads initially to a boat form which can undergo conformational inversion to the equatorial α-bromoketone. The alternative mode of attack in which bromine attacks from the opposite face (antiparallel attack) leads directly to the axial α-bromoketone. In the absence of strong interactions this mode of attack prevails.

The intervention of steric factors can be seen in the kinetically controlled bromination of steroidal 3-ketones. Bromination of 5α-cholestan-3-one or 3-acetoxy-5α-cholest-2-ene under kinetic conditions affords almost entirely 2α-bromo-5α-cholestan-3-one. However, in the 19-nor series in which not only are both the Δ^2- and Δ^3-enolates produced but also antiparallel attack is no longer hindered by a 1:3-diaxial methyl interaction, the axial (β) products are obtained. Thus bromination of 19-nor-5α-androstan-3-one gives a mixture of 2β-bromo-5α-androstan-3-one (63%) and 4β-bromo-5α-androstan-3-one (37%). However, where two enol-acetates are produced the relative proportions of each isomer can depend upon the reaction conditions. Furthermore, kinetically controlled bromination, even by operating in the presence of a base such as pyridine, is susceptible to the detail of the reagent. Hence the stereochemical consequences of the kinetic products are not fully clarified.

Under more acidic conditions a third feature, namely the thermodynamic control of the reaction, has to be taken into account. In particular a number of hydrogen bromide catalysed isomerizations are known. These can involve either the migration of a bromine atom to a less substituted carbon atom (e.g. 5α $\rightarrow$ 7α, 9α $\rightarrow$ 12α, 8β $\rightarrow$ 6α, 2,2 $\rightarrow$ 2α, 4α) or inversion to the more-stable isomer (e.g. 6β $\rightarrow$ 6α). In these subsequent isomerization reactions the configuration of the bromine atom is determined as a result of competition between the carbonyl and C$-$Br dipole interactions and steric interactions. The influence of ring junction on bromination can be seen in the bromination of 5β-cholestan-3-one which forms 4β-bromo-5β-cholestan-3-one.

(f) *Photochemical substitution reactions*

In recent years the activation of the angular methyl groups, particularly at C-19, by transannular photochemical substitution reactions has become important in the production of 19-nor steroids. Essentially these reactions depend upon the generation of an oxygen radical by photolytic cleavage of chlorite, hypoiodite or nitrite esters. When this radical is in the proximity of a hydrogen atom which it may abstract preferably through a six-membered transition state, a carbon radical is generated. This may recombine with the acyl fragment to form an alkyl iodide, or C-nitroso compound. The former can readily give a cyclic ether or undergo further substitution with the eventual formation of a lactone whilst the latter tautomerizes to an oxime. These reactions are summarized in Table 2.

TABLE 2. TRANSANNULAR PHOTOCHEMICAL REACTIONS

Functional group	Reagent	Product
OH CH$_3$ (C–C bridged by C)	I$_2$/Pb(OAc)$_4$ hν	O——CH$_2$ (C–C bridged by C)
OCl CH$_3$ (C–C bridged by C)	hν	O——C=O (C–C bridged by C)
ONO CH$_3$ (C–C bridged by C)	hν	OH CH=N·OH (C–C bridged by C)
CH$_3$NI CH$_3$ (C–C bridged by C)	hν	CH$_3$N——CH$_2$ (C–C bridged by C)
NH$_2$ CH$_3$ (C–C bridged by C, O= on left C)	I$_2$/Pb(OAc)$_4$ hν	O——CH$_2$ (C–C bridged by C, O= on left C)
N$_3$ CH$_3$ (C–C bridged by C, O= on left C)	hν	HN——CH$_2$ (C–C bridged by C, O= on left C)

In the steroid series the 1:3-diaxial relationship required for this reaction exists between an axial functional group at C-6 and the angular methyl (C-19). Oxidation of 6β-hydroxy steroids using iodine and lead tetraacetate gives a high yield of the 6β,19-ether, whilst 2β- and 4β-hydroxysteroids are converted to 2β,19 and 4β,19-hemiacetals. By making use of the 5α-halogeno-6β-hydroxy compounds (available from the addition of the hypohalous acid to a Δ^5-ene) a convenient synthesis of 19-nor steroids has been devised.

One of the most spectacular applications of nitrite photolysis is in the facile conversion of corticosterone acetate (20) to aldosterone acetate (21).

Corticosterone Acetate
20

Aldosterone Acetate
21

READING REFERENCES

Textbooks
E. L. ELIEL, N. L. ALLINGER, S. J. ANGYAL and G. A. MORRISON, *Conformational Analysis*, Interscience, London, 1965.
M. HANACK, *Conformation Theory*, Academic Press, London, 1965.
G. H. WHITHAM, *Alicyclic Chemistry*, Oldbourne Press, London, 1965.
P. B. DE LA MARE and W. KLYNE, *Progress in Stereochemistry*, Vols. 1-3, Butterworths, 1954–62.

Review articles
D. H. R. BARTON and R. C. COOKSON, *Quart. Rev.* **10**, 44 (1956).
D. H. R. BARTON and G. A. MORRISON, *Fortschr. Chem. Org. Naturstoffe* **19**, 165 (1961).
J. McKENNA, R.I.C. Lecture Series, 1966, No. 1.

CHAPTER 4

Molecular Rearrangements of Steroids

THE steroidal skeleton undergoes a number of rearrangements under acidic, basic and photolytic conditions. Although the outcome of these rearrangements depends upon the conditions, the site and conformation of the leaving group and the possibility of neighbouring group participation, nevertheless certain generalizations are possible. Firstly an equatorial leaving group facilitates ring contraction whilst an axial leaving group facilitates the migration of substituents as in a 1:2-shift. For example, dehydration of 3β-hydroxy-4,4-dimethyl cholestane (1) with phosphorus pentachloride gives *inter alia* the A-nor steroid (2) whilst dehydration of the corresponding 3α-(axial) epimer (3) leads to 3,4-dimethyl-cholest-3-ene

(4) by migration of a methyl group. Secondly, acid-catalysed carbonium ion rearrangements tend to proceed in the direction of the more highly substituted ions, a feature illustrated above. Accompanying this is the obvious tendency to diminish steric interactions.

In this discussion we shall describe acid-catalysed re-arrangements first followed by base-catalysed and then photolytic transformations.

4.1. ACID-CATALYSED REARRANGEMENTS

The importance of the stereochemistry of the system in determining a $1:2$-shift is well illustrated by the dehydration of the 5α-alcohol (5) to give a compound which is the acetate of "Westphalen's diol" (6). In this it can be seen that the departing hydroxyl group, the migrating methyl group and the hydrogen atom which is lost as a proton, each possesses a *trans* diaxial relationship to the other. However, more subtle features must also contribute to the reaction. Although, for example, it does not occur in the absence of a 6β-acetoxyl group or when the 5α-hydroxyl is alkylated or acetylated, a similar rearrangement is observed during dehydration of 4β-, $5\alpha,7\beta$-trihydroxycholestane-$4\beta,7\beta$-diacetate.

The formation of Westphalen's diol is an example of the more general class of "backbone" rearrangement. These rearrangements can also be initiated by the boron trifluoride-catalysed cleavage of $5:6$-epoxides. These products represent a further series of hydride and methyl shifts eventually leading to a compound such as (7). An interesting aspect of this rearrangement occurs in the 3-oxo-4,4-dimethyl steroid series in which cleavage of the $5\beta,6\beta$-epoxide leads to "backbone" rearrangement by migration of the β-C-19-methyl group. On the other hand, rearrangement of the 5α-epoxide led to a spiran (8). A consideration of molecular models might lead to the opposite conclusion, namely that cleavage of the 5α-epoxide should lead to methyl migration.

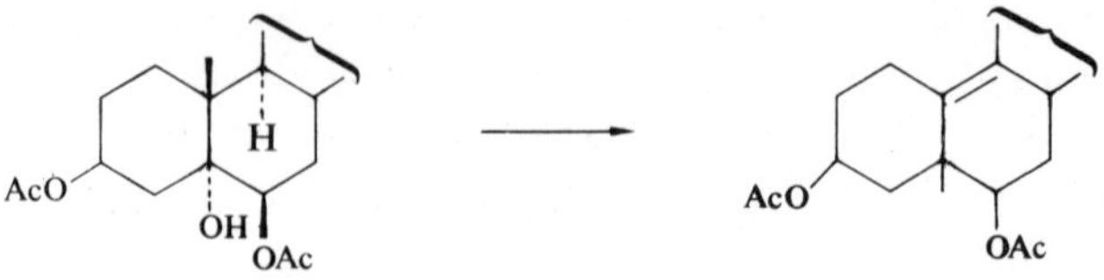

5

6

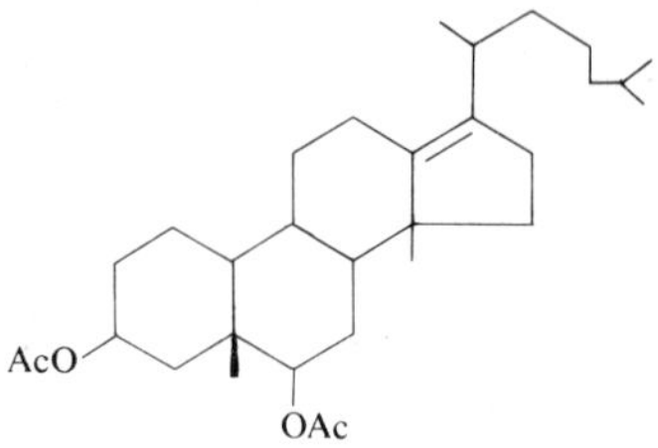

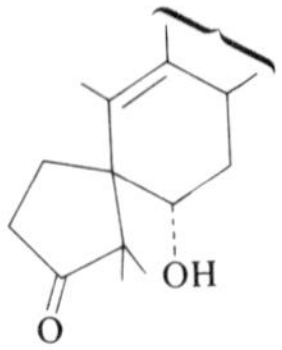

7

8

We have already noted that elimination of 3β-substituents can, in the case of the 4:4-dimethyl steroids, lead to ring-contraction. In the presence of a Δ⁵-double bond the reaction takes a different path. Thus hydrolysis of cholesteryl tosylate (9) in aqueous acetone containing potassium acetate gave a 3:5-cyclosteroid known as *i*-cholesterol (10). The location of the hydroxyl function at position 6 in this product was established by the identity of the corresponding ketone with that produced by reacting 3β-chlorocholestan-6-one with strong base. The solvolysis is unimolecular and proceeds through the formation of a homoallylic bridged cation. As a consequence of this not only is the reaction stereospecific with respect to 3β-substituents but also cleavage of the cyclopropane ring leads to 3β-substituted steroids. Thus reverse rearrangement with zinc acetate in acetic acid leads to cholesteryl acetate. Furthermore, solvolysis of the toluene-*p*-sulphonate of 3β-hydroxymethyl-A-norcholest-5-ene gives the same alcohols obtained from cholesteryl toluene-*p*-

sulphonate indicating the formation of the same non-classical carbonium ion (12). In contrast to this the toluene-*p*-sulphonate of 3α-hydroxymethyl-A-norcholest-5-ene (13) affords 3β,5-cyclo-5β-cholestan-6β-ol (15), which arises from a different cationic intermediate (14).

The formation of similar cyclo steroids have been noted in other cases. On the other hand, attempts to replicate the *i*-steroid rearrangement with pseudocholesterol (Δ^4-cholesten-7-ol) were unsuccessful.

The rearrangement of cross-conjugated dienones to phenols has been examined in the steroid series. The intervention of a spirocyclic intermediate, which was first substantiated in model studies by Woodward, has been confirmed with the rearrangement of steroidal 1,4-dien-3-ones. Thus androstan-1,4-diene-3,17-dione (17) gives the *p*-phenol (16) with anhydrous acid in acetic anhydride and the *m*-phenol (18) with aqueous mineral acid. The rearrangement of the dienone is probably initiated by protonation of the carbonyl group. The cation so formed can rearrange through a spiran intermediate (19) to the *p*-phenol (16). Alternatively a single methyl migration leads to the *m*-phenol (17). The related dienol-benzene rearrangement has been observed in treatment of 3β-hydroxy-androst-1,4-dienes with acid. Again a spiro-cation is envisaged as an intermediate. Some aspects of the mechanism have received support from tracer studies using 1-dehydro-[4-^{14}C]-testosterone and locating the final site of radioactivity in the product.

Although not related to this mechanistically the angular methyl group of the dienone (17) is extruded as its anion by

the action of lithium and biphenyl to give a derivative of oestrone. An interesting example of this rearrangement is shown by the conversion of the ether (20) to the phenolic ether (21).

4.2. BASE-CATALYSED REARRANGEMENTS

A number of ring contraction and expansion reactions arise through the action of base. They may be classified on the basis of oxidation level of the starting material, i.e. the re-arrangement of derivatives of (i) an alcohol; (ii) a glycol; (iii) an α-ketol; (iv) an α-diketone.

An example of the first class is found in the rearrangement on solvolysis of the equatorial 12β-mesylate of rockogenin (22) to form the C-ring contracted substance (23) possessing a carbon skeleton similar to that found in the alkaloid jervine.

A similar rearrangement occurs in the alkaline decompos-ition of the toluene-p-sulphonylhydrazone of hecogenin. Ring contraction of ring C can proceed in another manner with the extrusion of a carbon atom. On refluxing the 11α-acetoxy-12β-mesyloxy compound (24) with 10% sodium methoxide in methanol, the aldehyde (25) was formed. In this reaction the migrating 9 : 11-bond is *trans*-anti-parallel to the equatorial leaving group. The corresponding 11α-mesyloxy-12β-acetoxy compound possesses a similar arrangement and also undergoes this rearrangement.

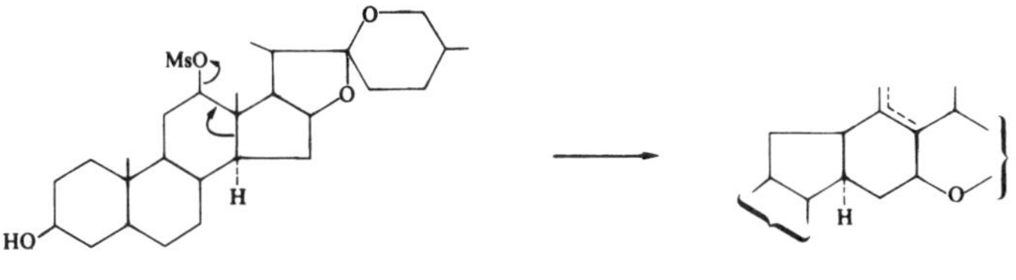

22

23

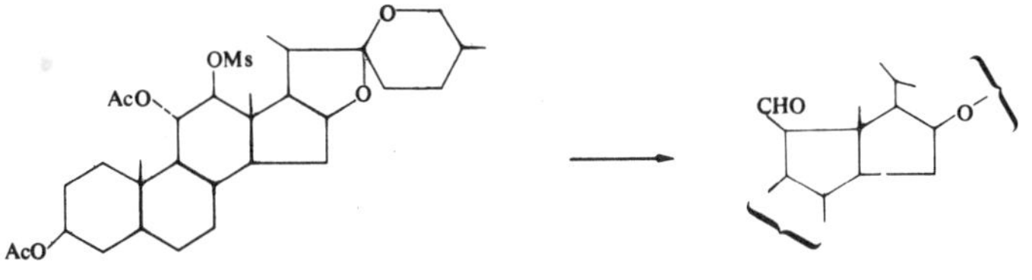

24

25

The $9\alpha,10\alpha$-diol (26) obtained by osmium tetroxide oxidation of Westphalen's diketone undergoes an interesting retroaldol and recyclization reaction. In the presence of mild base the *cis* fused isomer (27) is formed whilst under vigorous conditions the phenol (28), which arises from the alternative mode of cyclization, is formed.

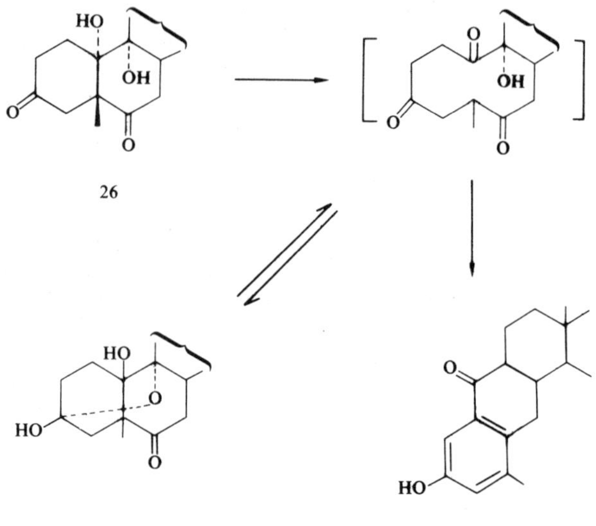

26

27

28

The third oxidation level represents that of the acyloin rearrangements. A number of examples of this are found in the steroid series. Thus reduction of 5α-hydroxycholestan-6-one with sodium and propanol leads to a mixture of cholestan-$5\alpha,6\alpha$-diol and cholestan-$5\beta,6\alpha$-diol. The latter is formed by the initial equilibration of the 5α-hydroxy-6-keto steroid with the corresponding 5β-hydroxy-6-keto steroid, by a reversible acyloin reaction (29–30).

29   30

31   32

The Favorski rearrangement of α-bromoketones involves the same oxidation level. Here displacement of the bromine atom with or without intervention of a cyclopropane intermediate leads to the formation of a carboxylic acid. This reaction has been applied in the contraction of both rings A and B. An example is found in treatment of the 7-bromo derivative (31) with triethylamine leading to the hydroxy-acid (32).

The benzylic acid rearrangement of steroidal diones represents the fourth oxidation level. In the majority of cases it has been used as a route to the nor-steroid. For example, cholestan-2,3-dione on treatment with potassium hydroxide in refluxing propanol gives an almost quantitative yield of the α-hydroxy acid (33) which is in turn oxidized to the A-norketone (34).

33   34

A number of ring contraction and expansion reactions are subject to both acid and base catalysis. An example of this is found in the acyloin rearrangements of 17-hydroxy-20-keto steroids. In the case of the 17α-hydroxy-20-keto steroids the action of base leads to the formation of 17-ketones. In strong base the formation of the anion (35) leads to a *trans* orientation of the carbonyl group and thus the stereochemistry (36) for the rearrangement product. In weaker base hydrogen-bonding prevails to orient the carbonyl *cis* to the 17α-hydroxyl (37) resulting in the opposite stereochemistry at 17a (38). In the presence of Lewis acids a co-ordinated complex is formed holding the carbonyl oxygen in the *cis* orientation. However, then the alternative migration (39) of the 14,17-bond occurs to give the 17a-ketone (40).

4.3. PHOTOCHEMICAL REARRANGEMENTS

The rearrangements described so far have been the consequence of either acidic or basic reaction conditions. However, a number of photochemical rearrangements exist in the steroid series some of which are of considerable importance. One chromophore is the carbonyl group. Irradiation of steroidal ketones can give a number of products. For example, the product of irradiation of androsterone is its 13-epimer, lumiandrosterone, formed by cleavage and recombination of the bond between the α-carbon atom and the carbonyl group. An alternative reaction, observed in reactive solvents such as methanol or water, is solvolysis of the diradical formed in this cleavage. Other examples of this reaction are found in the 3:4-cleavage of ring A of the triterpenoids during the partial synthesis of dihydronyctanthic acid and in the elucidation of the structure of dammarenolic acid.

Irradiation of ketones can also lead to the abstraction of an appropriately situated γ-hydrogen atom. The diradical which is formed can then breakdown as in the mass spectrometer or they may recombine to form a cyclobutanol. For example, 3,3-dimethoxypregnan-20-one (41) gives the cyclobutanols (42). Other aspects of this type of abstraction reaction which

41

42

43

44

can lead to photochemical substitution as in the photolysis of nitrites, have been described earlier. Ring contraction may occur on irradiation of α-diazoketones. This sequence has been used in the formation of a four-membered ring D (e.g. 43–44).

A number of photochemical rearrangements involve electron redistribution within a cyclic conjugated system. Some of these may be summarized by the generalization due to Barton.

The photochemistry of ergosterol to give the vitamin D precursor precalciferol, represents an important example of this cleavage. These thermal and photochemical reactions can be rationalized in terms of the Woodward–Hoffman rules, namely that polyolefins with $(4n+2)$ electrons cyclize and are formed thermally in a disrotatory manner and photochemically in a conrotatory manner whilst the reverse holds for systems with $4n$ electrons. Thus precalciferol (45) with $(4n+2)$ electrons cyclizes under thermal conditions to give the *cis* fused isopyrocalciferol (46) and pyrocalciferol (47). Under photolytic conditions ergosterol (48) and lumisterol (49) are formed. The sigmatropic 1:7-hydride transfer in the conversion of precalciferol to calciferol (50) involves a hydride transfer which, in order to maintain orbital symmetry, must involve a twisted transition state with transfer to the opposite face of the molecules.

Precalciferol   Isopyrocalciferol   Pyrocalciferol
45   46   47

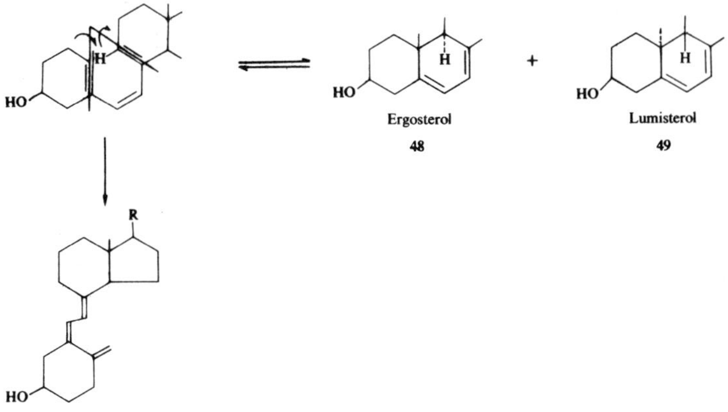

Ergosterol
48

Lumisterol
49

Calciferol
50

Irradiation of heteroannular dienes has been the subject of less-intense study. Thus irradiation of cholesta-3,5-diene gives the 3β-5 cyclosteroid (51) with the opposite stereochemistry to the product of the *i*-steroid rearrangement.

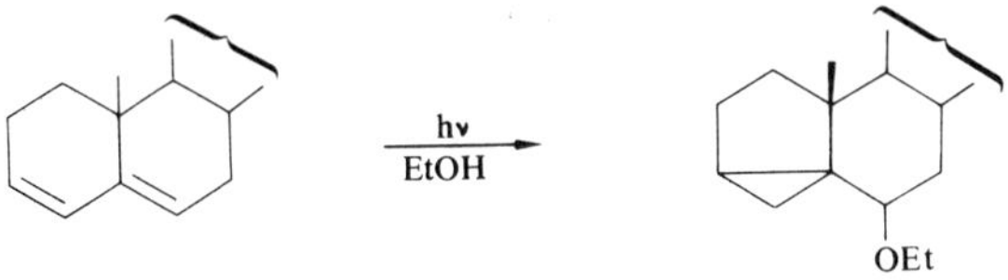

$\dfrac{hv}{\text{EtOH}}$

OEt

51

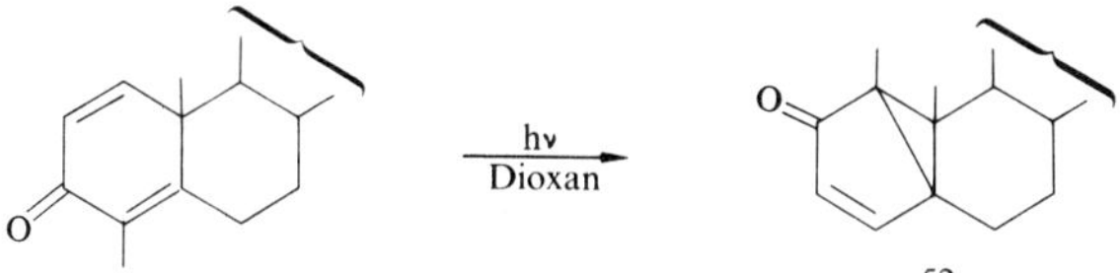

$\dfrac{hv}{\text{Dioxan}}$

52

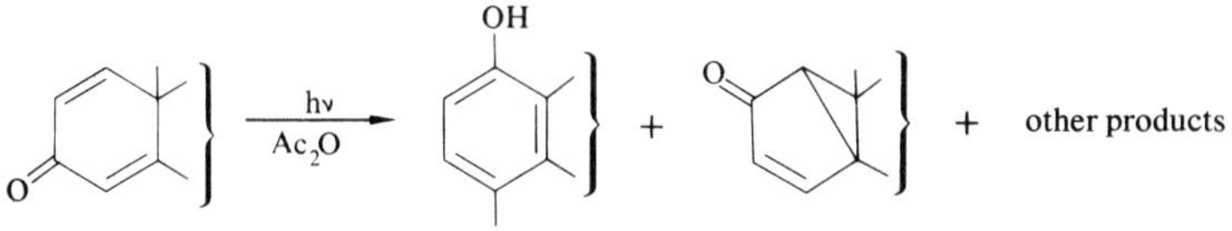

$\dfrac{hv}{\text{Ac}_2\text{O}}$

OH

53

54

+   other products

The photochemistry of cross-conjugated dienones, originally investigated in the chemistry of santonin, has been studied in the steroid series. However, the results are more complex. Irradiation of 1,2-dehydro-4-methyltestosterone acetate in dioxan gives mainly the cyclopropyl ketone (52). On the other hand, irradiation of 1,2-dehydrotestosterone acetate in acetic anhydride leads to a wide range of products. Some of these (e.g. 54) arise in a similar manner to the cyclopropyl ketone (52) whilst others such as (53) appear to be photochemical analogues of the dienone-phenol rearrangement.

READING REFERENCES

Textbooks

P. DE MAYO, *Molecular Rearrangements*, Vols. I and II, Interscience, London, 1963.

Review articles

P. DE MAYO, in BENTLEY and WEISSBERGER, *Structural Elucidation of Natural Products*, Interscience, 1963.

P. DE MAYO and S. T. REID, *Quart. Rev.* **15**, 393 (1961).

R. N. WARRENER and J. B. BREMNER, *Rev. Pure and Appl. Chem.* **16**, 117 (1966).

CHAPTER 5

The Synthesis of the Steroids

STEROID synthesis has been the object of many studies since the correct structure of cholesterol was proposed in 1932. The importance of the steroids in medicine has given a marked impetus to this work. Its development has been intimately linked to the increasing knowledge of the stereochemical consequences of synthetic reactions. In cholesterol there are eight centres of asymmetry thus giving 256 possible stereoisomers. In other terms as far as the carbon skeleton is concerned some sixteen carbon–carbon bonds have to be formed with the correct stereochemistry. However, not all these problems needed to be surmounted at once and there exist steroids with fewer asymmetric centres.

The first synthesis, that of equilenin (1), was described by Bachmann and Wilds in 1939. Oestrone (2) contains two further asymmetric centres. A total synthesis of oestrone was reported by Anner and Miescher in 1947 and this was followed by other successful syntheses by W. S. Johnson. However, the synthesis of the non-aromatic steroids represented a much more formidable task. Two different syntheses were announced in 1951. One was the Cornforth–Robinson synthesis from Oxford and the other by R. B. Woodward from Harvard. Subsequent years have seen the publication of about twenty-five syntheses including that of cortisone in 1953 and aldosterone in 1957. Each of these is distinguished by specific stereochemical features. However, it is not our plan to review each one in detail. Rather we shall select specific synthetic problems and illustrate the ways in which they were overcome. The problems resolve themselves into two main classes. The first involves the construction of the overall carbon skeleton and the second is concerned with the stereospecific introduction of functionality at particular sites on the carbon skeleton with the object of producing biologically active steroids. Although obviously the results overlap, one is essentially the total synthesis of the steroids and the other that of the partial synthesis of rare steroids from relatively abundant naturally occurring material.

5.1. RING-FORMATION REACTIONS

The various total syntheses that have been described are classified in terms of the order in which the rings are added. Thus the synthesis of equilenin mentioned above which involved the sequential addition of the rings, is described as $AB \rightarrow ABC \rightarrow ABCD$. Most of the early syntheses were linear schemes whilst some of the more recent syntheses have employed convergent schemes in which, for example, rings A and B and ring D are formed separately and then linked to form the ABCD system. This latter method has obvious economic advantages. The stereoselectivity of the reactions available now permit the total synthesis of steroid hormones on the industrial scale using a convergent scheme of this type.

A number of general reactions have been used for ring syntheses. One of the most important of these is the "Robinson ring-extension" reaction. Essentially this reaction involves the Michael addition of an enolate ion to an alkyl vinyl ketone to form a 1:5-diketone. Under the basic conditions of the reaction this is then cyclized to form a cyclohexenone. The reaction is exemplified in (3), an important stage in the Oxford synthesis.

Other examples of this type of addition involve the use of acrylonitrile in Woodward's total synthesis as in (4), The use of a protecting group, in this case the methylanilino-methylene grouping, directed cyanoethylation to the required tertiary centre.

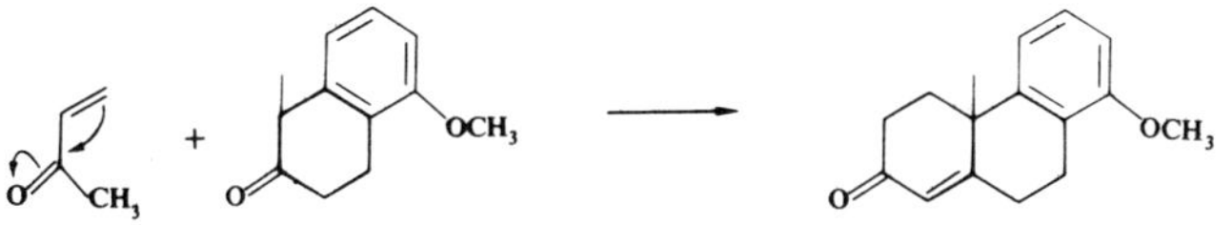

3

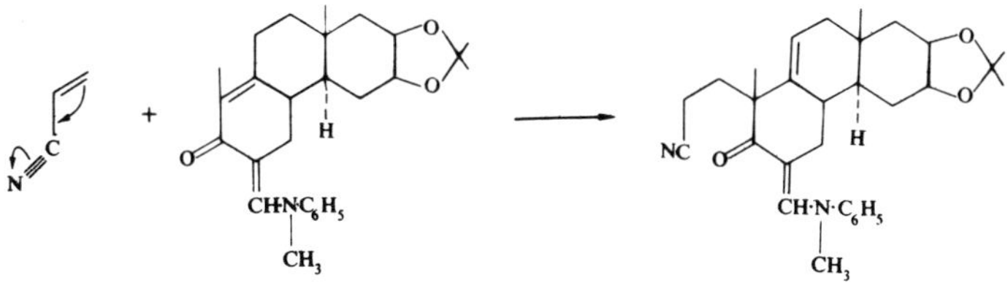

4

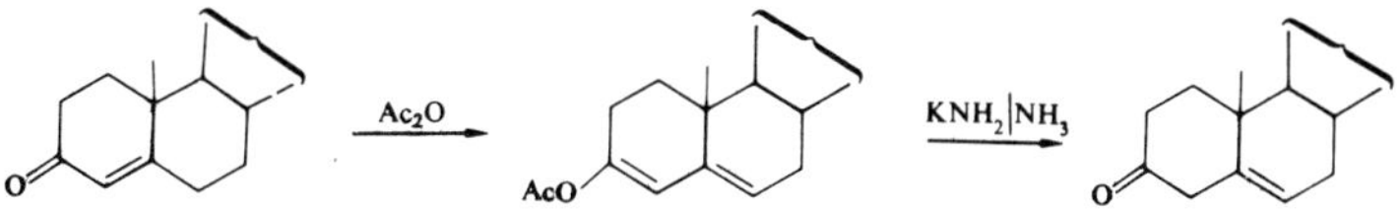

5

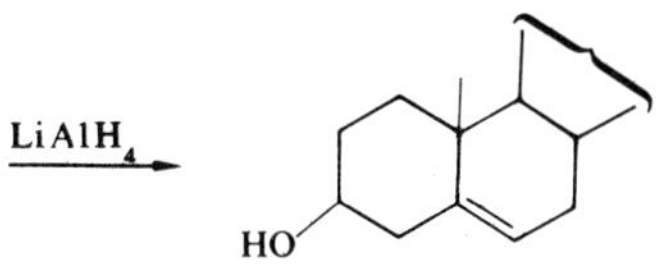

6

An important feature of the Robinson ring-extension reaction and its relatives is that it introduces a double bond at a ring junction permitting subsequent control over the ring-junction stereochemistry on reduction. Alternatively by the reaction sequence (5) to (6), the Δ^5-system of cholesterol may be produced.

An alternative reaction sequence involves the use of the Diels–Alder reaction. However, this leads to a *cis*-fused ring junction. Nevertheless, by using a *p*-benzoquinone as the dienophile, the product then possesses a carbonyl adjacent to the ring junction thereby permitting subsequent epimerization to the *trans*-fused system. This approach (7) provided rings C and D of the Woodward synthesis. In some instances a *cis*-fused system is an advantage in subsequent steps. For example, a *cis*-fused decalin produced by the sequence (8) was used in the Merck cortosone synthesis. The *cis*-fused B/C system was used to direct the stereochemistry of the formation of ring A.

7

8

The Dieckmann cyclization of esters has been used in a number of syntheses. The formation of the angularly alkylated *trans*-fused hydrindane belonging to rings C and D has been one of the problems of steroid synthesis.

Its solution in the first successful synthesis of equilenin involved the cyclization of the diester (9) with methoxide. Another interesting application came in a synthesis of oestrone developed by W. S. Johnson in 1951. The trimethyl ester (11) produced by a Stobbe condensation of (10) with methyl succinate, was cyclized to (12). This cyclohexanone (12) possesses its substituents in equatorial conformations.

The acid-catalysed cyclizations of olefins appeared from model examples to afford little control over the stereochemistry of the final ring junctions. However, recently the demonstration of the intervention of squalene epoxide in the biosynthesis of lanosterol and hence the steroids, has led to a renewal of interest in this approach. In model studies it has been possible to obtain a good degree of stereospecificity in the cyclization of (13) to (14).

The acid-catalysed alkylation and acylation of aromatic rings provides a means of constructing the polycyclic steroid ring system particularly as methods exist for the reduction of phenol ethers. Furthermore, a number of important steroids exist in which ring A is aromatic. Most syntheses involving substitution at an aromatic centre employ an anisole as the aromatic component. In these cases attack is directed primarily to the activated para position. The aromatic ring may then be reduced by a metal-amine solution. An example of this type of reaction is found in a recent remarkably short synthesis of (±)-oestrone. The vinyl ketone (15) is reacted under mildly basic conditions with 2-methylcyclopentane-1,3-dione to form the trione (16) in the first stage of a Robinson ring-extension reaction. The trione is subjected to cyclodehydration with polyphosphoric acid to form (17). By catalytic and then lithium, aniline-liquid ammonia reduction, this is converted to oestrone. There is an 18% overall yield from 3-*m*-methoxy-phenylpropyl bromide which served as the starting material for the synthesis of the vinyl ketone.

5.2. CONTROL OF RING JUNCTION STEREOCHEMISTRY

When a ring junction is formed under equilibrating conditions the *trans* isomer often predominates. Under other conditions in which the *cis* isomer is formed appropriate steps have to be taken for its subsequent isomerization. Other methods involve the protection of the ring junction by a double bond. The subsequent conversion of an sp^2 carbon to an sp^3 carbon of the correct stereochemistry then presents a stereochemical problem. Catalytic reduction can be particularly sensitive to stereochemical control. Thus in the reduction of a Δ^5 olefin the angular methyl group directs addition to a *trans* A/B fusion.

The Birch reduction of both aromatic systems and $\alpha\beta$-unsaturated ketones has a number of applications in this context. The reduction of unsaturated systems by a dissolving metal reagent in a sequence which involves the formation of a carbanion at a ring junction usually results in the formation of the thermodynamically more stable isomer. The most impressive application of this reagent in steroid synthesis comes in the synthesis of ($\pm$)-epiandrosterone by W. S. Johnson. Reduction of (20) leads to a 25% yield of a mixture (21) in turn hydrogenated to (22). The synthesis of the unsaturated intermediate (20) involved two ring-extension reactions. Thus the methoxy-β-tetralone (18) was condensed with the vinyl ketone derived from 1-diethylamino-3-pentanone methiodide to form the tricyclic ketone (19) which was then subjected to a second ring-extension reaction to form the tetracyclic ketone (20). This sequence illustrates the simplicity with which a tetracyclic skeleton can be constructed.

5.3. SELECTIVE ALKYLATIONS ·

The methyl groups of the steroid nucleus are sited at angular positions. Various methods of controlled alkylation have been developed to direct alkylation at these sites. For example, the angular position of a decalone (23) can be alkylated after the methylene position has been blocked either through the formation of a benzylidene derivative or a vinylamine derivative (24). The latter sequence involves condensation with ethyl formate to give a hydroxymethylene compound which is then reacted with N-methylaniline to form the vinylamine (24). Alkylation with methyl iodide and potassamide then takes place at the angular position. The protecting groups may be removed by successive acid and alkaline hydrolysis.

23   24

An indanone gives the more stable *cis* isomer under these conditions. Therefore the chrysene approach, involving alkylation of a six-membered ring D, was used to overcome this difficulty. Unfortunately alkylation of this particular system (22) is directed by the other angular methyl group to give a greater proportion of the unwanted α-methyl isomer. In this instance the furfurylidene protecting group was used to facilitate the subsequent cleavage of ring D with ozone to a dicarboxylic acid. This was cyclized to give ($\pm$)-epiandrosterone (25). It has been observed that introduction of a $9:11$ double bond, however, favours *trans*-alkylation of the C/D ring junction presumably by altering the transannular interactions in the transition state. An example of the use of this chrysene approach is found in a total synthesis of oestrone. The adduct of the diene (26) and benzoquinone was reduced to the diketone (27). This formed a mono-ketal (28) which on Wolff–Kishner reduction and epimerization at C-14 afforded the mono-ketone (29). Alkylation of the furfurylidene derivative gave a preponderance of the desired C/D *trans* methylated product (30). Cleavage of ring D gave (±)-homomarrianolic acid methyl ether (31) which had in turn been converted to oestrone (32).

5.4. PARTIAL SYNTHESIS OF STEROIDAL HORMONES

The application of steroid hormones and their analogues in therapy has led to the development of a number of partial syntheses of the relatively rare hormones from more abundant starting materials. The bile acids, such as cholic acid and deoxycholic acid, form one source of starting material whilst the sapogenins such as diosgenin (33) form another. A number of stages in these partial syntheses can be discerned although the order in which these are followed varies according to the specific objective. Thus the first stage involves the modification of the side-chain to form the pregnane skeleton. This in turn is converted to the androstane series or to the adrenocortical hormones. Modification of the functional groups on the ring system may then be carried out.

5.5. THE PARTIAL SYNTHESIS OF THE PREGNANE SERIES

Diosgenin (33) forms a readily available starting material obtained from Mexican Dioscorea species. Acetolysis leads to cleavage of the spiroketal system and the formation of a pseudosapogenin diacetate (34). Chromium trioxide oxidation of this cleaves the enol-ether of the side-chain to form the keto-ester (35). Elimination of the ester then leads to 16-dehydropregnenolone acetate (36). The pregnane side-chain can be eliminated by a number of oxidative procedures. Alternatively, conversion to the oxime (37) followed by Beckmann rearrangement affords the enamine acetate (38) which is hydrolysed to the 17-ketone (39), thus providing a convenient route to the androstane series.

Removal of the side-chain of the cholic acid series follows a modification of the Barbier–Wieland degradation due to Meystre and Miescher. The diphenylethylene (41) which results from the reaction of the bile acid ester (40) with phenyl magnesium bromide and dehydration, is brominated with

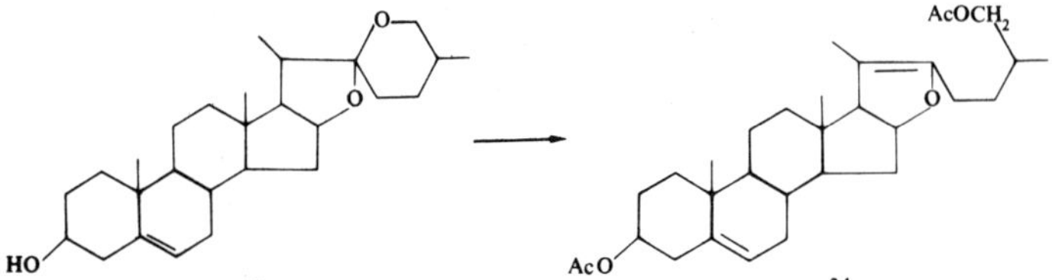

33

34

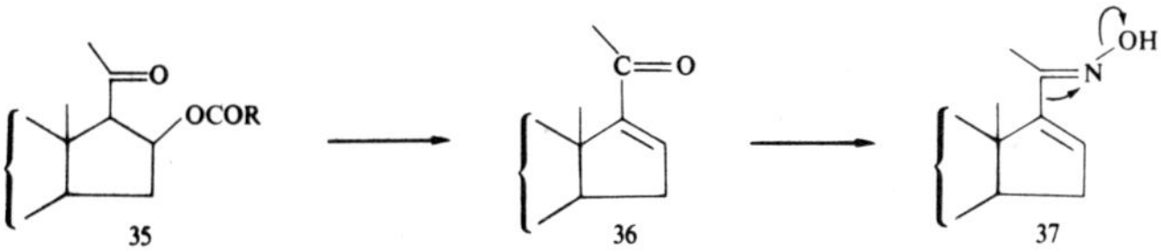

35

36

37

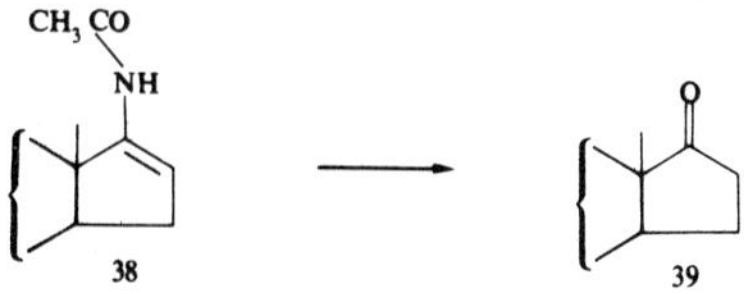

38

39

N-bromosuccinimide to give the allylic bromide. Dehydro-halogenation affords the diene (42) which is oxidized with chromic acid to form a 20-ketone (43). This procedure was employed in a partial synthesis of progesterone from 3β-hydroxy-Δ^5-cholenic acid.

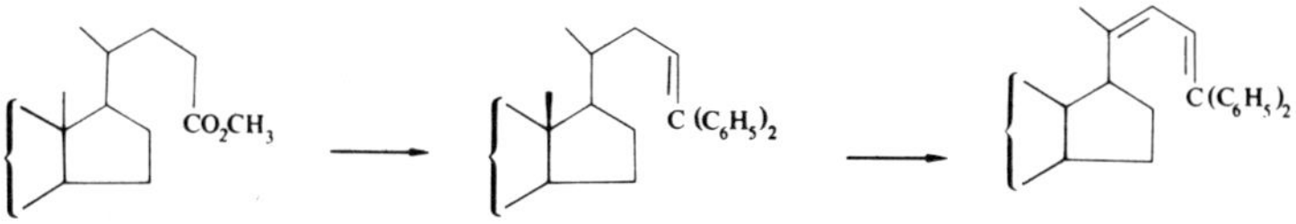

40

41

42

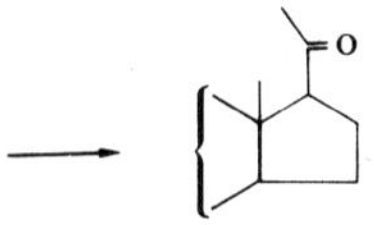

43

5.6. PARTIAL SYNTHESIS OF THE
ADRENOCORTICAL HORMONES

The features that need to be introduced into the steroid framework are: (a) an oxygen function at C-11; (b) the dihydroxyacetone side-chain; (c) a ring A $\alpha\beta$-unsaturated ketone-Δ^4-3-one; (d) various additional substituents such as a 9α-fluoro group, and a 16α-alcohol which contribute to increased therapeutic activity.

Steroids with an oxygen function at C-11 are relatively rare and hence a number of methods were developed to introduce functionality at that site. Selective reactions were facilitated by the steric hindrance at the 11-position. One method involves the transfer of an oxygen from C-12 to C-11. The bile acid, deoxycholic acid (44) ($3\alpha,12\alpha$-dihydroxy-5β-cholanic acid), was used in the first investigations of this route. Subsequently the sisal sapogenin, hecogenin (45), has been employed. Pyrolysis of 12α-benzoates led to an 11-olefin

(46). Addition of hypobromous acid gave the bromohydrin (47) which was in turn oxidized to the 11-ketone. The 12α-bromine was reductively eliminated with zinc and acetic acid. An alternative procedure involved bromination of a 12-ketone. The product (48) underwent hydrolysis and isomerization to the 11-keto-12-ol. Deacetoxylation of the corresponding 12-acetate with calcium in liquid ammonia furnished a route to the 11-ketone. Another process involved as one step the displacement of an allylic 12α-halogen (49) with 3α:9-ether formation (50). Subsequent modification of the double bond permitted the introduction of oxygen at C-11 and the cleavage of the ether ring.

A number of routes involved dehydrogenation of compounds containing a 7-ene to form the 7:9(11)-dienes. Further oxidation of these gave, for example, the Δ^8-7,11-enedione. Conversion to an 11-ketone involved reduction to the 7,11-dione with zinc and acetic acid followed by selective Wolff-Kishner reduction of the 7-ketone.

Commercially one of the most important methods involves microbiological hydroxylation. Many fungi are capable of stereospecifically hydroxylating steroidal substrates in high yield. In 1952 it was found that *Rhizopus arrhizus* and *R. nigricans* were capable of converting progesterone to 11α-hydroxyprogesterone in high yield. *Aspergillus niger* and *Cunninghamella blakesleana* are also used for microbiological transformations. There are now reports of hydroxylation at most sites on the steroid framework.

A number of routes have been developed for the elaboration of the characteristic dihydroxy-acetone side-chain. Reaction of 17-ketone (51) with potassium acetylide gives an ethynyl alcohol (52). Attack occurs from the α-face of the molecule to give 17β-alcohol. Partial hydrogenation gives an olefin which undergoes allylic rearrangement to the primary acetate (53). Hydroxylation of the 17–20-olefin with osmium tetroxide gives the 21-acetate of a 17α,20β,21-triol in turn oxidized to a 20-ketone (54). An interesting method of introducing a 17α-hydroxyl in the pregnane side-chain (55) involves enol-acetylation to give a 17–20-enol acetate (56). Epoxydation of the olefin followed by treatment of the oxide with acid to give a 17α-hydroxy-20-ketone (57). Alternatively bromination and dehydrobromination of a 20-ketone gives a 16-olefin. Epoxydation and reductive opening of the 16α,17α-epoxy-20-ketone leads to the 17α-hydroxy-20-ketone.

The generation of Δ^4-en-3-one forms the final stages of several partial syntheses. Even in cases in which the system is generated early in a synthesis it is protected during subsequent manipulation. Oppenauer oxidation of a Δ^5-3-alcohol, as found in cholesterol and in compounds derived from 16α,17α-oxide of dehydropregnenolone, results in the Δ^4-3-

one. An alternative method involves bromination and dehydro-bromination of a 3-ketone.

The application of cortisone to the treatment of the rheumatoid arthritis is accompanied by the appearance of various side effects. Hence various modifications of the natural steroids have been made with objective of increased activity and the elimination of undesirable side effects. Thus introduction of a 9α-fluorine enhances anti-inflammatory activity but further modification was required to eliminate undesirable mineral corticoid effects. The 1-dehydro derivative of cortisone, prednisone, produced by microbiological dehydrogenation is valuable in this respect. Further improvement was found in the introduction of a 16α-hydroxyl group. Combination of these three features led to the analogue triamcinolone (58) which possesses high glucocorticoid and anti-inflammatory properties and is almost free from salt-retaining properties.

58

Further modifications of this structure by the formation of a 16α,17α-acetonide and the introduction of a 6α-fluorine have led to further improvement. Other modifications have involved the introduction of 16α-methyl group.

READING REFERENCES

Review articles

J. W. CORNFORTH, *Progress in Organic Chemistry* 3, 1 (1955).

L. VELLUZ, J. VALLS and G. NOMINE, *Angew. Chem.* (Internat. Ed.) 4, 181 (1965).

CHAPTER 6

The Biosynthesis of the Steroids

THE detailed studies of cholesterol biosynthesis, particularly through the work of Bloch, Cornforth and Popjak, and Lynen, have resulted in a clarification of the essential features of this pathway. Further studies on steroid metabolism have served to indicate the relationship of the classes of steroid to each other. Cholesterol (5) is terpenoid in origin, i.e. it is a compound in whose biosynthesis isopentenyl pyrophosphate (1) forms an

The stages in cholesterol biosynthesis

irreversible intermediate. Six units of isopentenyl pyrophosphate are utilized in this process which involves the formation of a triterpene, lanosterol (4) and the subsequent loss of three methyl groups. For the purpose of this description we will discuss the biosynthesis in the following stages: (i) the conversion of acetate to isopentenyl pyrophosphate and the head-to-tail polymerization of three of these units to yield farnesyl pyrophosphate (2); (ii) the dimerization of two farnesyl units to form squalene (3); (iii) the cyclization of squalene to lanosterol (4) and its conversion to cholesterol (5).

6.1. THE CONVERSION OF ACETATE TO ISOPENTENYL PYROPHOSPHATE AND FARNESYL PYROPHOSPHATE

Observations on the incorporation of acetate labelled in the methyl group with deuterium and on the carboxyl group with ^{13}C suggested that this two-carbon unit formed a primary precursor of cholesterol. Indeed in 1937 in one of the earliest applications of isotopic labelling to biosynthetic problems, trideuteroacetic acid, was fed to yeast cells and the resultant yeast sterol was found to contain a large amount of deuterium. However, it was not until the post-war years that the distribution pattern of the acetate units was completely worked out with ^{14}C by a series of degradations which involved the identification of the origin of each carbon atom. These results are summarized in (6).

6

The methods that were used may be exemplified by the isolation of ring A. Cholest-5-ene (7) on ozonolysis formed a keto-aldehyde which was cyclized to the B-nor aldehyde (8). Further ozonolysis of this and decarboxylation of the resultant pyruvic acid gave a 1 : 5-keto-aldehyde (9). This underwent a retro-Michael reaction with the separation of ring A as 2-methylcyclohexanone which was further degraded.

These studies by Bloch and by Cornforth and Popjak showed that the methyl and carboxyl carbon atoms alternate in the carbon skeleton of cholesterol whilst the pendant carbon atoms arise exclusively from the methyl group of acetic acid. A distribution of this kind suggested that the C-5 terpene unit was formed from three molecules of acetic acid by way of acetoacetate and a C-6 unit such as β-hydroxy-β-methyl glutaric acid.

The fortuitous discovery of mevalonic acid (10) as an essential growth factor for *Lactobacillus acidophilus* at a time in which a number of five- and six-carbon units were being screened as steroid precursors enabled rapid progress to be made. In 1956 Tavormina, Gibbs and Huff were able to show that cell-free extracts from liver were able to incorporate radioactively labelled mevalonic acid into cholesterol. One enantiomorph of ($\pm$)-mevalonic acid was required for the biosynthesis. Furthermore, it was established, using [1-^{14}C]-mevalonate, that the carboxyl group was lost during biosynthesis.

Cell-free extracts from yeast and liver were utilized in the study of the biosynthesis of squalene from mevalonic acid. Adenosine triphosphate, Mg^{2+} ions and TPNH were essential for biosynthesis. The conversion of mevalonic acid to isopentenyl pyrophosphate involves the stepwise ATP dependent phosphorylation to form successively the 5-monophosphate, the 5-pyrophosphate and finally a 3:5-phosphorylated intermediate. The latter undergoes ready decarboxylation and elimination to form isopentenyl pyrophosphate (11). This intermediate was isolated by the addition of an enzyme inhibitor, iodoacetamide. Isopentenyl pyrophosphate forms a mandatory intermediate in terpene biosynthesis.

The intervention of farnesyl pyrophosphate in the biosynthesis of squalene was demonstrated by omitting TPNH from the cell-free enzyme system used in the conversion of mevalonic acid to squalene. Under these conditions farnesyl pyrophosphate accumulated. The first step in the conversion of isopentenyl pyrophosphate to farnesyl pyrophosphate was shown to be its enzymic isomerization to dimethylallylpyrophosphate (12)−a reaction inhibited by iodoacetamide. This unit formed the terminal isopropylidene group of farnesyl pyrophosphate. Geranyl pyrophosphate and farnesyl pyrophosphate have been identified as precursors of squalene in yeast systems. The condensation of dimethylallylpyrophosphate with isopentenyl pyrophosphate to form geranyl pyrophosphate (13), and of geranyl pyrophosphate with isopentenyl phrophosphate to form farnesyl pyrophosphate involves the elimination of the allylic pyrophosphate possibly through the intervention of an allylic cation, although a concerted process is clearly possible (12). By using stereo-specifically deuterated mevalonic acids (prepared by reduction

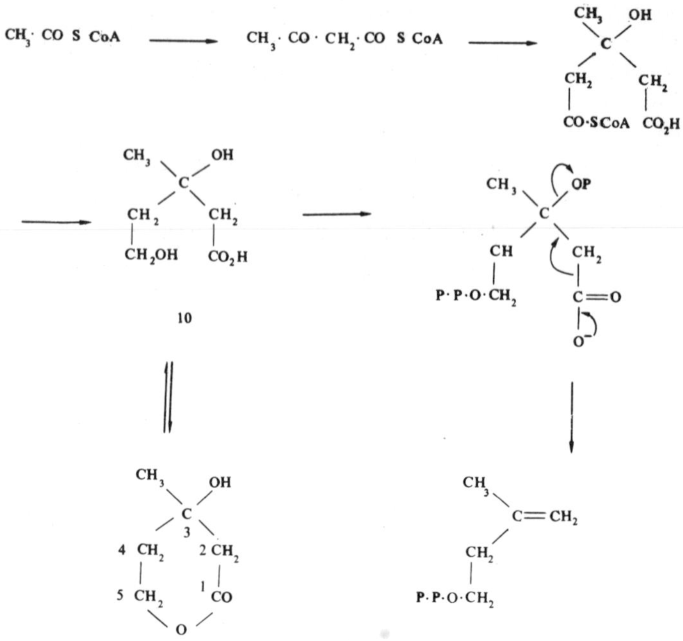

CH₃·CO S CoA ⟶ CH₃·CO·CH₂·CO S CoA ⟶

Formation of Isopentenyl Pyrophosphate
SCoA = Co-enzyme A., P.P. = pyrophosphate

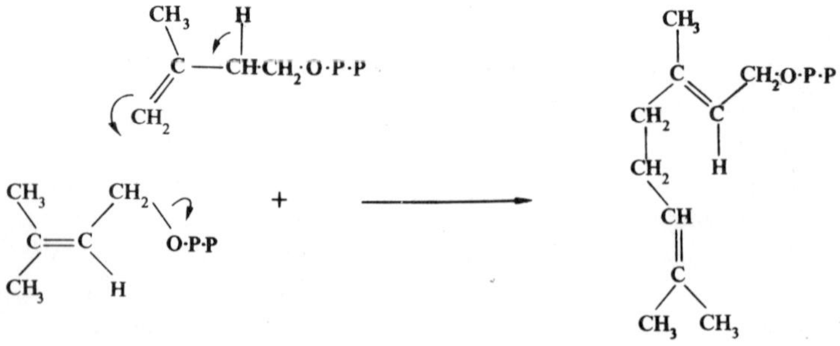

10

11

12

13

of mevaldic acid with $NADH^2$) inversion was shown to take place at C-1 of the dimethyl allylpyrophosphate in a manner consistent with a bimolecular nucleophilic substitution.

6.2. THE DIMERIZATION OF FARNESYL PYROPHOSPHATE

When radioactive farnesyl pyrophosphate was incubated with yeast enzymes and TPNH, radioactive squalene was formed. Two units of the pyrophosphate condense in a head-to-head manner with the formation of squalene. However, when squalene was synthesized from mevalonic acid labelled with deuterium at the 5-position, eleven of the possible twelve deuterium atoms were retained. A detailed mass-spectrometric study of the degradation products of squalene showed that a deuterium atom is lost from the central two carbon fragment of squalene. The origin of the incoming hydrogen atom was shown to be NADPH. Furthermore, this process was shown to be stereospecific by isolation of the trideuterosuccinic acid from this central fragment and demonstration of its optical activity. By using stereospecifically mono-deuterated meva-lonic acids it was possible to generate *in situ* stereospecifically labelled farnesyl pyrophosphate and hence squalene. Examination of the optical activity of the dideuterosuccinic acid representing the four middle carbon atoms of squalene showed that the overall process involved in the combination of two farnesyl pyrophosphate resulted in retention of configuration at C_1 of one molecule and inversion at the other.

Several mechanisms have been proposed to account for this. One involves isomerization of farnesyl pyrophosphate to nerolidyl pyrophosphate which then condenses with the second molecule, anchimeric assistance being provided by the terti-ary pyrophosphate. Elimination and subsequent reductive elimination of the cyclic phosphate results in the formation of squalene bearing one central hydrogen of non-mevalonoid origin. A second mechanism invokes the formation of a farnesyl

-S-enzyme complex. Alkylation on sulphur by a second farnesyl pyrophosphate leads to a sulphonium salt capable of undergoing a Stevens rearrangement. Reductive displacement of the sulphur enzyme then leads to squalene.

Two possible mechanisms for the coupling of Farnesyl Pyrophosphate

6.3. THE CONVERSION OF SQUALENE TO LANOSTEROL

The intervention of squalene and lanosterol in cholesterol biosynthesis has been shown in a number of systems. During the conversion of squalene to lanosterol a rearrangement of the methyl groups at the centre of the molecule is involved. Labelling experiments indicate that this involves two 1 : 2-shifts.

The nature of the cyclizing agent has been the subject of speculation. Oxygen from $^{18}O_2$ but not from H_2O^{18} was incorporated into lanosterol and hence species such as OH^+ were invoked.

However, recently squalene mono-epoxide (15) has been shown to be very efficiently converted by rat-liver system to lanosterol and the steroids. During this cyclization the methyl groups of the terminal isopropylidene groups of squalene retain their individuality. Thus in the cyclic soyasapogenol only one of these groups is labelled, by [2-^{14}C]-mevalonate. The extra side-chain methylene of ergosterol and eburicoic acid is then introduced at this stage from the methyl group of methionine.

The conversion of lanosterol to cholesterol involves the sequential loss of three methyl groups, the migration of the Δ^8 double bond to Δ^5 and the reduction of the side-chain. A number of stages in this conversion involving the oxidation of the methyl groups and their elimination as carbon dioxide have been established. Thus there is evidence for the intervention 4,4'-dimethylcholesta-8,24-dien-3β-ol (17) in this process and it seems likely that the further loss of methyl groups takes place in a stepwise fashion.

The C_{27}-steroid resulting from the demethylation of lanosterol (16) is cholesta-8,24-dienol (15) known as zymosterol. The conversion to cholesterol involves reduction of the side-chain double bond and rearrangement of the nuclear double bond. This rearrangement is dependent on oxygen and the process appears to involve isomerization to Δ^7-cholestenol,

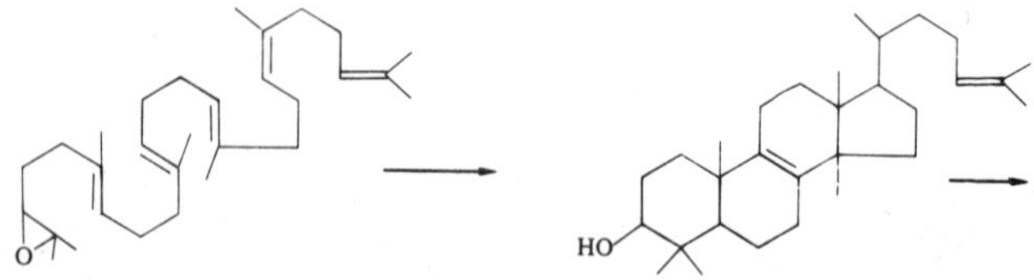

15

16

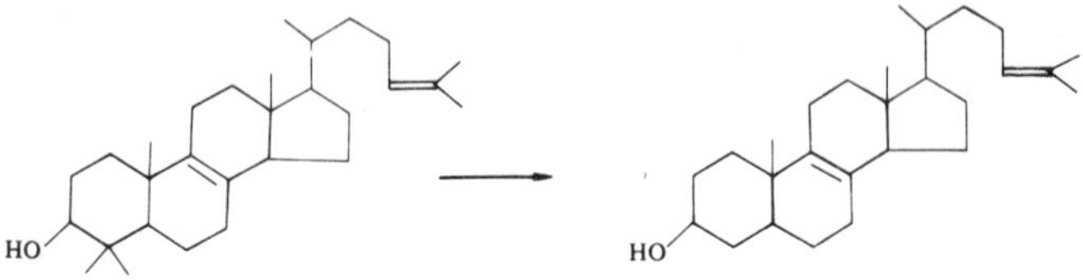

17

18

oxidation to 7-dehydrocholesterol and finally reduction to cholesterol. Cholesterol occupies a central position in the biosynthesis of many other steroids. Thus it has been shown to be converted to the bile-acids such as cholic acid. In this biosynthesis it would appear that the appropriate nuclear transformations, such as hydroxylations and reduction of the double bond, take place prior to cleavage of the side-chain. On the other hand, the formation of the steroid hormones involves cleavage of the side-chain to form pregnenolone, the remaining carbon atoms appearing as isocaproic aldehyde. Further conversion of pregnenolone can lead to androsterone or by successive hydroxylation and oxidation to the cortico-steroids.

READING REFERENCES

Textbooks

CIBA Foundation Symposium: *Biosynthesis of Terpenes and Sterols*, ed. WOLSTENHOLME and O'CONNOR, Churchill, London, 1959.

J. H. RICHARDS and J. B. HENDRICKSON, *The Biosynthesis of Terpenes, Steroids and Acetogenins*, W. A. Benjamin, New York, 1964.

R. I. DORFMAN, *Metabolism of Steroid Hormones*, Academic Press, New York, 1965.

Review articles
R. B. CLAYTON, *Quart. Rev.* **19**, 168; 201 (1965).
J. W. CORNFORTH and G. POPJAK, *Advances in Enzymol.* **22**, 281 (1960).

Index